Competing with the Sylph

Competing with the Sylph

Dancers and the Pursuit of the Ideal Body Form

L. M. Vincent, M.D.

Andrews and McMeel, Inc.
A Universal Press Syndicate Company
Kansas City · New York · Washington

Library of Congress Cataloging in Publication Data

Vincent, L   M
   Competing with the Sylph.

   Includes bibliographical references.
   1. Ballet dancing—Physiological aspects.
2. Women dancers—Diseases and hygiene.
3. Reducing—Physiological aspects. 4. Ballet
dancing—Psychological aspects. 5. Women—
Physiology. I. Title.

RC1220.B27V56   613'.04'24   79-20501
ISBN 0-8362-2405-1
ISBN 0-8362-2407-8 **pbk.**

For my parents and sister,
on our anniversary

Contents

Acknowledgments

Now, anxious to allow my typewriter the privacy of its own case, I am able to offer only the humblest of thanks to those largely responsible for what I place my own name upon.

First, to the many professional dancers, students, instructors, and administrators, for their cooperation and candor, as well as to the following group of professionals, consultants who provided their experience, expertise, feedback, and suggestions: Richard M. Bachrach, D.O. (Osteopathy); David V. Forrest, M.D. (Psychiatry); Rose E. Frisch, Ph.D. (Public Health); David M. Garner, Ph.D. (Psychology); William G. Hamilton, M.D. (Orthopedics); Jack Katz, M.D. (Psychiatry); Barnard Kleiger, M.D. (Orthopedics); Edith J. Langner, M.D. (Endocrinology); Ernest Leibov, M.D. (Psychiatry); William A. Liebler, M.D. (Orthopedics); Eugene L. Lowenkopf, M.D. (Psychiatry); Alan H. Pressman (Chiropractic); Mona Shangold, M.D. (Gynecology); Robert A. Vigersky, M.D. (Endocrinology); Michelle P. Warren, M.D. (Gynecology); and Barnett Zumoff, M.D. (Endocrinology).

Clive Barnes, Alexandra Danilova, Iris Fanger, Anna Kisselgoff, John Gruen, and Marcia Siegel were generous in sharing their time and special perspectives on dance.

Robert P. Hudson, M.D., and Bernice Jackson hospitably coordinated my excursions through the Logan Clendening History of Medicine Library at the University of Kansas Medical Center.

Arthur R. Clemett, M.D., arranged the necessary time flexibility for the project, and Jim Andrews, my publisher, once again let himself be convinced.

Bill Batson and Jim Goss provided photographic services and were fortunate enough to have Flora Ann Hall for their subject.

And finally, I am obliged to David F. White, Mark Shwayder, Robert N. Reeves III, and S. L. Hearing, who provided the advice and support that comes only with friendship.

Introduction

Life is short, and the art long; the
occasion fleeting; experience fallacious,
and judgment difficult.
　　　—Hippocrates, First Aphorism

As a lover of the dance, I am vulnerable to its mystique. Truthfully, I'm all for the mystique, and would hope to be blinded by it completely for the two hours or so that I'm seated upon a red velour cushion in the first ring of the New York State Theater. But I would also hope to control that mystique somewhat, just as a rheostat connected to an electric light may modulate the gradations from a full intensity of wattage to a barely discernible amber. For most of us, the artistic sensibility must be brightened and dimmed according to things of this world, mundane things such as muscles and tendons, hormones and blood sugar levels, anxieties and dreams.

Certainly the mystique will wax and wane for the dancer, whether he or she be motivated by necessity, love, an inner need or compulsion, or a spark of magic. What is evoked upon a stage may be illusive, but the sweat, dedication, denial, and pain are very real. There is nothing mystical about not having enough weeks of performing to be eligible for unemployment. There is nothing mystical about an injury that threatens a career for which a twenty-three-year-old has strived for as long as she can remember. There is nothing in the least mystical about continually having to confront one's failures. The life of a dancer may or may not be rewarding, but most assuredly it will not be easy.

Throughout my exposure to and association with the dance world, I accepted certain aspects of the subculture as "part and parcel" of dancing. My medical bent was directed primarily toward physical injuries encountered by dancers, generally problems of an orthopedic nature. There was a security in such a narrow focus; troublesome considerations outside of the specific domain could be justifiably cast aside, taken for granted as part of a framework within which one must of necessity operate. But then the lighting changed. Vividly I recall the specific moment when I became conscious of a different angle of vision.

While walking down Sixth Avenue I passed a young ballet scholarship student from a company ballet school. I had seen her and others like her many times before, on my daily jaunts to and from the hospital. Hair pulled severely and pinned into a chignon, she walked turned-out; wore a bulky sweater, jeans, and clogs; and carried an overstuffed dance bag by a strap across her shoulder. On that particular day I did not see a starry-eyed ballet student coming from her adagio class; I saw a pale, gaunt seventeen-year-old with dark circles under her eyes and a downcast gaze. Her unhealthy visage bore none of the physical exuberance and vitality usually associated with exercise. She looked terrible.

As it happens, she had danced seven hours that day and had eaten only an orange and a slice of mango. Later I also learned that she had been inducing vomiting on a regular basis for three months in an effort to attain her "ideal" dancing weight. Concern with weight and diet, with looking like a ballerina—one of those idiosyncrasies that are "part and parcel" of the dance world—had become a vicious, self-destructive obsession.

To assume that artistic considerations are in any way linked to health considerations is totally unrealistic and naive. A choreographer, for example, may be at liberty to manifest concern for a dancer only insofar as that person conforms to his artistic vision; maintenance and preservation of health need not be the top priority. Individuals are not only forgotten with the passage of time; in some circumstances they are expendable commodities in the present.

This is not to suggest that artists should have the sensibilities of doctors, or vice versa, a swap that might just result in riveting dialogue among physicians, but would undoubtedly mean pretty lousy art for everybody else. The point is that much of the responsibility for good health always rests with the individual. But paradoxically, in our "health-conscious" society, ill-advised health practices continue to abound, the result of exploitation, ignorance, and the sacrifice of common sense to a variety of dictates that may in themselves be distorted and arbitrary.

Whether one is a fashion model, a housewife, an athlete, or a blue-collar worker, one is likely to be victimized to some extent by a culture obsessed with thinness, youth, and beauty. While dancers are not alone in the not infrequent bartering of their physical well-being, by focusing our gaze upon them we can see quite clearly how difficulties ranging from poor weight control to menstrual dysfunction may be both self-inflicted and self-perpetuated.

One cannot consider health in its broadest sense without an awareness of its setting; the values and assumptions implicit in a particular social context provide a useful perspective on "why," rather than "how," difficulties may arise. Thus, I concern myself here with more than matters strictly medical and depart substantially from the constraints of standard scientific writing in the hope of conveying a "feel" for the subculture that serves as a model. I have attempted, then, to integrate current medical knowledge, as it relates specifically to the health of dancers, from a variety of disciplines in a manner both palatable and comprehensible to those for whom it is directly or indirectly pertinent.

Casting the mystique completely by the wayside, I will admit that—given the choice—I appreciate the beauty of a well-functioning, healthy body more than the beauty of a ballet line. In the sense that this is a subjective judgment, my perspective is slightly biased. However, did I feel in the slightest degree that the two were mutually exclusive, I never would have embarked on the writing of this book.

L. M. Vincent, M.D.
Kansas City/New York City

Competing with the Sylph

Before the Mirror

THE SUBCULTURE: GENERALIZATIONS AND BIASES

For quite some time, a six-pack of Tab sat untouched on the bottom shelf of my refrigerator, reminding me of the perils of stereotyping.

Now I don't particularly care for Tab, but after months of interviewing dancers, I had become somewhat habituated to the subtleties of the subculture. I had grown accustomed to feeling gluttonous as I stretched my masseter muscles around an overstuffed pastrami sandwich while a dancer sat demurely nearby, daintily spooning up yogurt or nibbling on some fruit or greens. In fact, I have to strain my memory to conjure the image of a ballet dancer drinking regular cola or using granulated sugar in tea or coffee (some would use honey). What echoes in my mind is the simple request that invariably followed a coffee order: "Do you have Sweet 'n Low?"

Which explains why I bought the Tab. In preparation for an interview, I made a special effort to be hospitable and accommodating. Admittedly it was a bit presumptuous, not unlike stocking up on caviar and vodka for a Russian houseguest.

"Would you like a diet cola?" I offered.

When the dancer replied in the negative, I was noticeably taken aback. Perhaps she had heard wrong.

"It's *Tab*," I reiterated.

"No, thank you," said the dancer, "I brought my own."

And from a blue canvas dance bag she pulled out a Dr. Pepper. Sugar-free.

Nondancers have often commented to me that they are able to spot dancers walking down the street. One medical colleague perceived this as a brilliant clinical diagnosis, a stroke of deduction worthy of Sherlock Holmes, but in fact all of us carry the badges of our respective subcultures, showing by our clothes, mannerisms, or speech who and what we are. One would be hard-pressed to find a certified public accountant who wore her hair in a chignon, walked with external rotation of the hips (see figure 1), and carried a dance bag. Certainly one could predict the occupation of my medical friend from his white coat and its attendant paraphernalia, the Cross pen and pocket flashlight in one pocket and the stethoscope tucked into, but revealingly dangling from, another.

Dancers belong to a very special community. In the most important sense they are bound together by the common experience of dance itself: tradition, technique, discipline, purpose.[1] Whether separated by miles or by continents, dancers will do the same or similar exercises, hear much of the same music; each will know the feel of the wood floor, the pain of pushing for a bit more extension, the satisfaction of accomplishment, the frustration of failure. The experience transcends all levels of living. The hopeful may not yet know the curtain calls or applause bestowed upon the soloist, but both will sew elastic on their slippers, wash their tights in the sink, carry bandaids and lambswool, be annoyed if they find themselves opposite the break of the mirror in class, and probably use more acrylic floor wax on their pointe shoes than on their floors.[2]

The crux of many of the dilemmas of the professional dancer is the precariousness of being simultaneously athlete and interpretive artist. In terms of athletic performance demands, classical ballet has been ranked second out of sixty-one sports (right behind football).[3] But all dancers rank second in a different category—in percentage of unemployment in the labor force of writers, artists, and entertainers (right behind actors).[4] Few sports competitors (one thinks of gymnasts and figure skaters as exceptions) not only undergo rigorous, continual training from an early age onward, but also must conform to the aesthetic demands of a visual art form. Both the football defensive tackle defending the goal line and the tenor bellowing Puccini are allowed the freedom of resembling beer barrels.

The adoption of a dance life style may often be narrowing and restrictive, entailing sacrifices that the run-of-the-mill athlete need not make. Not only may the commitment to intensive

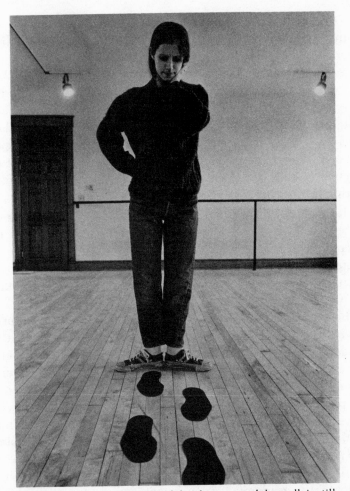

Figure 1: Take away the dance bag and the chignon, and the walk is still a dead giveaway. The walking apparatus of the ballet dancer is not mutated; rather the peculiar stride results from external rotation of the hips transplanted to the street. Disadvantages: 1) aesthetic considerations; 2) possible calamities on stairwells if not modified while wearing high-heels; 3) hindrance of maximum running velocity; 4) possible contribution to overstretching of the posterior tibiales tendons. Advantages: 1) comfort (force of habit); 2) badge of peer group identification, particularly for younger dancers; 3) ability to walk silently even when wearing corduroy pants.

(Photo by William H. Batson)

training begin at a young age, but for the most part that training is uninterrupted and often exclusive. Unlike the football or baseball player, the dancer has no off-season or spring training. From the fledgling to the famous, there is always the class, regardless of season, day in and day out. Agnes de Mille, like every other aspiring young dancer, quickly learned "the first all-important dictate of ballet dancing—never to miss the daily practice, hell or high water, sickness or health, never to miss the barre practice; to miss meals, sleep, rehearsals even but not the practice, not for one day ever under any circumstances, except on Sundays and during childbirth."[5]

Many professional athletes, as well as amateurs of Olympic caliber, acquire their training in conjunction with college (99 percent of NFL players, for example, played college ball), the military, or even a professional career outside of their athletic discipline. The classical ballet dancer will more likely be called upon to burn the bridge of higher formal education in the furtherance of her chosen field. Despite the growing number of university-affiliated dance programs, university graduates are by and large "too old" to be accepted by the major classical ballet companies. The dominating trend is for the youngster to develop and travel through the ranks of a performing arts school or a company school. Not uncommonly, young classical dancers who come to New York City from elsewhere finish high school in an accelerated, condensed program (four years into three), obtain high school equivalence by correspondence or proficiency exams, or forego the diploma altogether.

Not that an academic curriculum vitae is very meaningful for a dancer, but then a career in dance is not particularly noteworthy for job opportunities, financial security, or, perhaps most important, longevity. A football player's career days may be numbered (or curtailed early by injury), but the practical benefits of the professional game include high salaries, opportunities for off-season and postretirement employment, life insurance, major medical coverage and dental insurance, and a pension.[6] Contrast this with the not unusual case of a ballet soloist in her early thirties who faces the end of a "successful" career with little education, borderline financial status, no non-dance-related skills, and perhaps no family of her own. With respect to practical matters, giving a dance career the "hard sell" takes quite an imagination.

Within the dance subculture, individuals are subjected to variable influences, and dancers themselves may be likely to stress differences more than similarities. Just as all dancers are—or perceive the need to be—thinner than the average person, classical dancers must generally be the thinnest of all types of dancers. Dancers in the highly competitive major companies in New York are as a rule thinner than nonprofessionals, or than regional or European dancers. Modern and jazz dancers usually have more flexibility in their training; they may realistically begin dance studies at a later age than ballet dancers, and a successful career for them does not as often preclude higher education. As an illustration, consider a comparison of the educational status of the members of a ballet with that of the dancers in a modern company, both located in New York City and both internationally renowned. Of the ninety-member New York City Ballet, only five dancers have attended college, and all of these are male.[7] The situation is quite different in the Martha Graham Company. Ten of twelve females have attended college, and nine of eleven males have some college credit; of the remaining four company members, three are of European origin and have accomplished course work equivalent to early college level.[8]

Obviously a comparison of a thirty-year-old modern dancer in a company of twenty with an eighteen-year-old ballet dancer in a corps of fifty is not a fair one. One can easily discern, though, how dance stereotypes arise, particularly when they are colored by biases, rivalry, and chauvinism. One modern dancer with whom I spoke was quite harsh regarding her classical counterparts. Her basic argument was that ballet dancers "don't have other lives or well-formed personalities," possess a "herd instinct and mentality," and "wear blinders." When I gave equal time to a ballet dancer, she countered quite matter-of-factly with, "Everyone knows that modern dancers are just frustrated ballerinas." From my standpoint, the score is now tied. Whether there are more girls in ballet with blinders on than there are frustrated ballerinas in modern does not seem to me a fruitful subject for debate.

THE OBSESSION

No one is free who is a slave to the body.
—Seneca (ca. 4 B.C.–A.D. 65)

As regards weight, I divide female dancers into two groups. First, there are the so-called naturally thin women who maintain a svelte body line without worrying much about food intake. And then there is the vast majority. Aside from their common preoccupation with food, the members of the latter group also share a gut-felt resentment for the former. Some of the resentment is probably undeserved, since a good number of those envied struggle as much as the rest, but are just more discreet about it.

If obsession with fat is a national pastime, then surely dancers are Olympic contenders. One might argue that dancers talk about, refer to, or pine over food more than anything else, from the succinct, "I'm fat," to the more winsome, "I wish I could lose a pound from the weekend," to academic diatribes on dieting methods and physiology. But whether or not the words are spoken, there is always the mirror. Watch a dancer scrutinizing herself in the mirror, probing her stomach, hips, and thighs with her fingertips, appraising from various angles (sideways for the assessment of protruding mid-section or rear, head on for the hips and inner thigh, peeking over the shoulder for a glimpse at the breadth of the behind). In her eyes is the glitter of the true believer on a search-and-destroy mission; she's going after that fat with the furor and frenzy with which one pursues roaches in the kitchen. An eighteen-year-old ballet student describes the compulsion: "When I look into the mirror I get so distracted I can't even concentrate when I don't think I look halfway decent.

It's like going to work and not brushing your hair, looking sloppy. It's in the same category as wearing a clean leotard, pinning your leotard so the line looks good. It's presenting yourself."

Dancers are justifiably preoccupied with weight, and the subculture guarantees its own peer group pressure and reinforcement. The concern—subtly pervasive and unavoidable—starts from the first step into the dance studio. With some amusement, an ex-ballet dancer related to me how her son's first ballet class affected him. The nine-year-old, with one hour's immersion in the subculture, came home for dinner and refused his favorite dessert. He, like many other perceptive and impressionable initiates, began the ritual of dieting with his first plié.

> I never had a weight problem at all, but I got to New York—and I've always been slim—and the school never told me to lose weight . . . and all of a sudden, everyone else around me was on a diet to lose weight. And when I think about it now—for no apparent reason—I felt I had to, I had to go on a diet. I had to stop eating meat. I had to stop having ice cream or cookies whenever I felt like it, and I had to lose weight. When I really didn't but just because everybody else did.
> —Ballet company member, age twenty (5'7", 117 pounds)

Inseparable from the obsession is the fact that the weight standard for dancers is different from that set for most people, much leaner than that suggested in charts, and much lighter than the weight most women would see as a reasonable dieting goal. Nondancers thus often find dancers' weight complaints a bit hard to swallow. A five-foot-five-inch ballet dancer will bemoan her natural disposition to obesity, only to disclose that the most she's ever weighed is a paltry—though horrifying to her—112 pounds. Hearing this—both sympathy and empathy vanishing like a coin from a magician's palm—a 150-pound woman might have to combat her own natural disposition to stomp on the dancer's toes.

Obviously a dancer's weight must be considered in the

context of her profession. From the onset, dancers must conform to more stringent standards, operate with a different set of aesthetic rules, look through fat-colored lenses, so to speak. In a sense this is a deviation from generally accepted norms, but it is very much a reality in the dance world, and doctors who routinely see dancers treat it as such. A New York City physician is matter-of-fact on the subject: "I have two girls overweight by [the choreographer's] standards. Now they're not overweight by medical standards, but they are overweight by professional standards. I put them on diets." The dancers themselves accept the reality to such a degree that the abnormal becomes normal to them. As one company member puts it: "A lot of us here have been doing this for such a long time, and as far as, like other women would want to have breasts, and would want to have hips, and would want to have thighs, then all of a sudden you hear this girl saying, 'Oh, if only I could get rid of my breasts.' So in that case, you lose a vision of what a woman should look like. And you might see someone walking down the street who has a beautiful body for a normal person, and you would think, 'Oh, she looks a little heavy.'"

It takes all sizes and shapes to populate the world, and we seldom question the reality of thinness in dance. There are many reasons and justifications for slenderness, some better than others, but all in some way contributing to our current notion of what dancers are supposed to look like. The bottom line is undoubtedly aesthetic, and that's pretty hard to argue with. In the words of a dance instructor and choreographer: "I think a thinner body is more attractive to look at than one of those Rubenesque-looking numbers. But some people don't. But when it's in a pair of pink tights, and you have all those bulges coming out, then I think it should be kept at home."

Balanchine once stated that he likes long women for his choreography because he can "see more."[9] Whatever the artistic preferences, there just isn't much of a premium for obesity upon the dance stage.

Once the aesthetic criteria are established, practical and

technical matters come into play. A former principal ballerina finds that "the technical demands nowadays made of females are tremendous compared to what they were. We're working on a tremendously high level of refinement and technique, so we're looking for a body that can endure more, that looks better."

Professional demands include a pleasing line, a suitable appearance (or sometimes the ability to fit) in costumes, a weight that can be lifted (which depends upon the size and strength of available males), and usually a reasonable degree of uniformity (a six-footer in a line of five-footers is quite distracting). A former dancer gives yet another reason, not particularly either accurate or important, but nonetheless one of my favorites: "Photographs add seven pounds. On stage you always look fatter."

In any case, there are plenty of reasons why dancers have to be thin, should one bother to ask. But there are many reasons why the aesthetic considerations of dance should not be given carte blanche. The pertinent question is not why dancers "have" to be thin; rather, it is how thin is "thin"? As I mentioned, it is difficult to dispute an artistic judgment; yet there's substantial variation in the fine tuning of what we consider "fat" and what we see as "thin," all of which is inextricably tied up in what we refer to as "beauty." Not that I think there will be much of a market in the foreseeable future for obese ballet dancers; still, let us cast aside our biases (as well as our knowledge of the exigencies of the dance world today) and assume a broader perspective. We might benefit by recognizing the arbitrariness, and even folly, of any "ideal" concept of beauty. Aesthetic "fine tuning," in fact, may be quite coarse, and the establishment of any "ideal" rather presumptuous.

A CRASH COURSE IN BEAUTY

It is certainly not true that there is in the mind of man any universal standard of beauty with respect to the human body. It is, however, possible that certain tastes may in the course of time become in-

herited. . . . If all our women were to become as beautiful as the *Venus dé Medici,*
we should for a time be charmed; but we
should soon wish for variety; and as soon
as we had obtained variety, we should
wish to see certain characteristics a little
exaggerated beyond the existing inheri-
tance.
    —Charles Darwin, *The Origin of the Species*

By today's standards, Venus is a tad chunky, and a well-inten-
tioned friend might even advise her to enroll at Weight
Watchers. But consider another Venus (figure 2), this one of
Willendorf, the oldest known representation of the human form.
Discovered on the banks of the Danube, and dating back to the
Paleolithic period, this obese woman with enormous breasts,
protruding belly, and monolithic thighs exemplifies the taste for
epic dowdiness that persisted in the Neolithic period, prehistoric
Greece, Babylonia, and in Egyptian sculptures.

Whether fat women predominated or were deemed desirable,
or whether the obesity was an artistic convention symbolizing
abundance and fertility, we can't be completely sure. But we do
know that even today, in certain societies, obesity is much
admired, even to the extent of being considered a secondary
sexual characteristic. A fat body may have the connotation of a
strong body, and since only women of leisure can afford the
luxury of immobilization, overfed women represent the state of
being well-to-do, and hence, part of the "beautiful people." In
some cultures on the African continent, brides-to-be-actually go
through preparations of excessive fattening. The "coming out"
of these debutantes consists of "going into" special houses for
fattening, where they are secluded for periods ranging from
several weeks to years (depending on their wealth), not unlike
geese destined to donate their lives for pâté de foie gras.

Attitudes toward fat, in the most elemental sense, depend
upon the availability of food, upon whether nature smiles or
frowns as far as nutritional prosperity is concerned. From the
long-range historical standpoint, nature's disposition has been

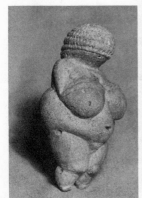
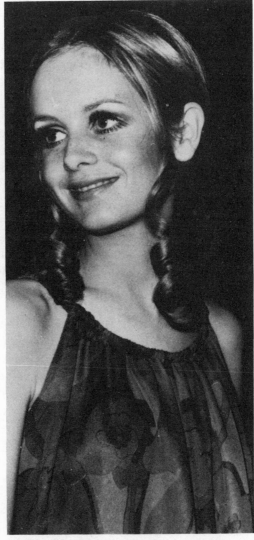

Figure 2: As an illustration that fashions change with the times (in this case, over a period of twenty thousand and some odd years), compare the somewhat different looks of the Venus of Willendorf (the stony-faced one on the left) and Twiggy (Lesley Hornby, circa 1967).
(Photos courtesy of Naturhistorisches Museum Wien and Wide World Photos)

quite sullen, if not downright vindictive. We do not usually ponder, as we weigh the merits of the spinach salad against those of the jarlsburg, avocado, and sprouts on whole wheat, the fact that for most of the people much of the time, the task has been much simpler—just to get enough of anything. Only when food is abundant can we indulge in gluttony and satiation or, even more important, afford the luxury of dieting and self-imposed starvation.

On this side of the body spectrum, various cultures have gone slightly overboard in their reaction against obesity. We know that the ancient Greeks envied their predecessors, the Cretans, who were supposed to have known of a drug that allowed them to eat all they wanted, yet remain thin. The Spartans as well as the Athenians were sticklers about fat (Socrates danced every morning to keep his figure), and the Roman ladies at the time of the empire evidently suffered to keep as slim as reeds. In the sixteenth century Montaigne wrote that women could swallow sand in order to ruin their stomachs and acquire a pale complexion.

In more modern times, a certain degree of indecisiveness has been the hallmark, with the pendulum swinging from one extreme to the other in periods of relatively (historically speaking) few years. At the turn of our present century, a buxom woman was in order. Consider the complaint of the French physician Heckel, who wrote the following in 1911:

> One must mention here that aesthetic errors of a worldly nature to which all women submit, may make them want to stay obese for reasons of fashionable appearance. It is beyond a doubt that in order to have an impressive décolleté each woman feels herself duty bound to be fat around the neck, over the clavicle and in her breasts. Now it happens that fat accumulates with greatest difficulty in these places, and one can be sure, even without examining such a woman, that the abdomen and the hips, and the lower members are hopelessly fat. As to treatment, one cannot obtain weight reduction of the abdomen without the woman sacrificing in her spirits the upper part of her body.

> To her it is a true sacrifice because she gives up what the
> world considers beautiful.[10]

In the twenties, a flat-chested, lean, and angular creature took
over. After another twenty years, the rotund look was again the
symbol of attractiveness. So when Twiggy hit the scene in the
mid-sixties (5'7", 92 pounds in her prime), exemplifying for
adolescents throughout the world what they might aspire to look
like when they "grew up," she represented merely another
variant of body overhauling in conformance to ever-changing
body ideals (see figure 2).

More disturbing than the mere arbitrariness of a beauty
concept are the awesome health consequences that previous
generations of women have had to endure. The attempt to
convert the female contour into an hourglass with the instrument
of torture known as the corset is an appropriate example. The
stout woman with the tiny waist—a species that had never before
existed in nature—evolved virtually overnight, thanks to the
crinoline corset reinforced with whalebone and steel ("tight
straps" were used earlier, but the more barbarous devices came
into vogue after 1854, with the whalebone variety marking an
advanced degree of female disfigurement). Women tolerated
and even sought a form of mutilation that reminds one of
foot-binding, a custom which persisted for over a thousand years
in China.

Aside from clawing the flesh and displacing internal organs
(the hazards of splitting steel stays were ever-present, particularly for those who exercised while corseted), the corset, through
pure mechanical pressure, undoubtedly decreased the volume of
food ingested, while serving at the same time as a strong
psychological inducement to further restrict intake. Even when
the harm of corsets had been recognized, the idiocy continued on
moral grounds, for an unlaced women had come to be regarded
as licentious, a veritable vessel of sin. One such symbol of
heresy, unlaced and barefooted, was Isadora Duncan, who
integrated an approach to dance with a crusade for corset
consumer protection. That women were eventually freed from

the grip, however, was probably not so much the result of Isadora's efforts as of good fortune thoroughly disguised. Only after the War Industries Board revealed that unbinding American women would release twenty-eight thousand tons of steel, enough to build two World War I battleships, did liberation from lacing hasten.[11]

A SOMEWHAT DIFFERENT LOOK AT "THE LOOK"

Bright little bird bones, delicate bird
sinews! She was all fire and steel wire.
There was not an ounce of spare flesh on
her skeleton and the life force used and
used her body until she died of the fever
of moving, gasping for breath, much too
young. . . . Her trunk was small and
stripped of all anatomy but the ciphers of
adolescence, her arms and legs relatively
long, the neck extraordinarily long and
mobile. . . . Without in any way being
sensual, being, in fact, almost sexless, she
suggested all exhilaration, gaity, and de-
light.
    —Agnes de Mille, *Dance to the Piper*

This twentieth-century description of Pavlova by Agnes de Mille might well be a voice from the nineteenth century preserved intact. More striking than the continued presence of Romantic ballets in modern repertory is the influence Romanticism has on our current concept of the "look" of the ballerina. Certainly the era of the Romantic Ballet must be seen in terms of the larger Romantic Movement in art and literature, and it was these times that gave birth to and nurtured the sylph. Representing lightness, ethereality, and spirituality, the sylph still connotes the "dreamy silhouette" to which many a ballet dancer may aspire. With a bit of medical-historical irreverence, we might examine the Romantic roots to illustrate why the sylph, not unlike the corseted woman, might have difficulty obtaining health insurance.

A perusal of a good part of the literature of the nineteenth century reads like copy for a cough syrup advertisement. Heroes and heroines hacked, shivered, chilled, coughed up blood, and fevered themselves into oblivion, albeit rather gracefully. Not that lung ailments, specifically tuberculosis (then called consumption), accounted for the Romantic Movement, but undoubtedly the disease contributed significantly to the gloom and weepiness that marked the tear-tracked face of the period. This mysterious affliction enlisted the greatest of sympathies and was a quite useful literary device—consumption was commonly believed to chiefly affect sensitive natures (it was once thought to enhance creativity). In addition, the tragedy of youth and beauty fading (". . . and the life force used and used her body until she died of the fever of moving, gasping for breath, much too young . . .") conferred a refined physical charm upon the stricken as they succumbed to a painless, poetical death. Before leaving this earth, one first had to go into decline, until substance gradually dissolved into spirituality, like houselights going into a slow fade.

Few diseases today have such positive connotations or artistic merit (one thinks of hypoglycemia, which is a bit trendy in dance circles, or perhaps various and sundry neuroses, pedestalized in the humor of Woody Allen). But tuberculosis was the darling of art and literature for half a century before losing its poetic luster, and it was, conveniently, as prevalent then as tendinitis is in dance classes or among joggers today. There were many notables who coughed, lay down, and were counted in the dismal parade of their art, among them several Brontës, Elizabeth Barrett Browning, John Keats, and Robert Louis Stevenson.

Aside from the creators themselves, models were similarly affected. Marguerite Gauthier, of *Camille* fame, was based upon Alphonsine Plessis, one-time mistress of Alexandre Dumas *fils,* a fashionable courtesan who led a whirlwind social life and was the center of worshipful attention wherever she went, until her death of consumption at age twenty-three. Mimi of *La Bohème* was in real life a flower girl in Paris who came to live with Henri Murger before also succumbing to the disease (Murger wrote *Scènes de la Vie de Bohème,* the basis for the Puccini opera). Janet

Burden and Elizabeth Siddal (married to Dante Gabriel Rosset-
ti), prominent models for Pre-Raphaelite paintings, were both
fragile, languishing, and long-limbed, and both, as unhealthy
symbols of the era, had tuberculosis.[12]

Thus, art imitated life, and life subsequently imitated the
imitation to mock itself, as ethereality became the vogue.
Observed Dumas: "In 1823 and 1824 it was the fashion to suffer
from the lungs; everybody was consumptive, poets especially; it
was good form to spit blood after each emotion that was at all
sensational, and to die before reaching the age of thirty."[13]

Paleness, not glowing health, was the fashionable attribute of
women, as men cultivated a passion for delicate, languishing
companions, threatened with impending death. The use of rouge
was abandoned in favor of the whitening powders. Regardless of
season, women were draped in various light materials, such as
unbleached batiste and embroidered organdy muslin. Weakness
and refinement became synonymous.

> The generation of 1830 liked its women to be charming,
> graceful, and delicate. It again became the fashion to be pale
> and to faint continually. . . . No women in society went
> without her lorgnette, which lent her an additional touch of
> amiable helplessness; and if she ate little at table, and put
> her glove by mistake into her glass, it all helped to show
> how ethereally she was constituted. . . . A woman who
> thought anything of herself could at the most allow herself
> to nibble a few sweetmeats; in 1825 she began to require
> water to rinse her mouth, and in 1830 bowls to wash her
> fingers in.[14]

The desire to appear pale was most assuredly not a particularly "healthy" impulse. Food habits, even among the prosper-
ous, were far from conducive to good health for a number of
reasons. Because of the obstacles of season and distribution, it
was not always an easy matter to get fresh milk and vegetables.
Also, there were certain prejudices against some types of food;
fear of typhoid and cholera, for example, contributed to the
avoidance of fresh fruits. At best, then, achieving adequate

nutrition was no mean feat, but compounded with the foolishness of fashion, it was a near impossibility. Young women took
to drinking lemon juice and vinegar as a means of killing their
appetite in order to attain the desired paleness. An 1824 article
called "Beauty Training for Ladies" recommended a diet which
prohibited all vegetables except potatoes, as well as butter,
cream, milk, cheese, and fish, all for the sake of the complexion[15]
(somewhat later, in the heyday of Victorianism, late nineteenth-
century women tended to eschew the same foods on moral
grounds; believing that foods from animals increased sexual
appetites).[16]

Thus, the real-life setting from which the sylph emerged in
ballet was amidst considerable coughing. *La Sylphide,* the first
ballet to reflect the characteristics of the Romantic Period,
premiered on March 12, 1832, with the title role danced by Maria
Taglioni. Significantly, this was one of the first occasions in
which a ballerina actually performed on her toes as opposed to
demipointe, enhancing the lightness and ethereality, shortening
the gap between the mortal and the supernatural. Of course, the
masterpiece which still serves as our example of the Romantic
Ballet surfaced nine years later with *Giselle,* in which the sylphs
were more specifically Wilis (spirits of betrothed girls who died
after being jilted; they dance their faithless lovers to death). The
libretto for the ballet was written by none other than Thèophile
Gautier, himself one of the leaders of the Romantic Movement,
who wrote of his youth: "I could not have accepted as a lyrical
poet anyone weighing more than ninety-nine pounds."[17]

Not that I am directly blaming Gautier for the current
popularity of Tab in dance circles. Nor am I suggesting that
Giselle really died of tuberculosis (though maybe she had a
touch of it—see figure 3). I have romped through the weed fields
of history only to illustrate that the rich ballet heritage includes a
tradition of fashion and beauty that is not exactly robust. Which
is why I cringe every time I hear mention of a "classical" ballet
body or the "striving for perfection." Perhaps I take these
phrases too literally, thinking back on the female of the

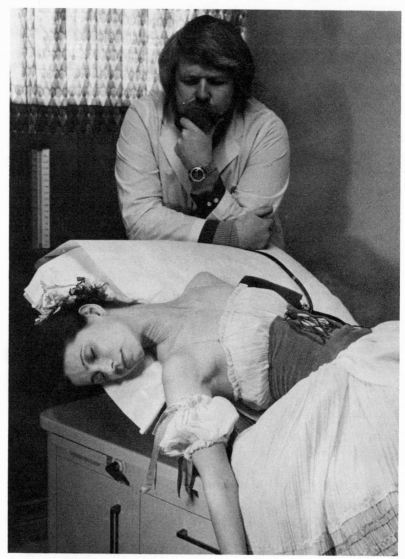

Figure 3: What really did Giselle in? Was it—as commonly believed—the result of a broken heart (secondary to adolescent adjustment reaction/hysterical personality), or did tuberculosis have something to do with it? Medical records are unavailable.
(Photo by L. M. Vincent)

nineteenth century slumped on her well-worn couch; for this young lady of good breeding has no ostensible appetite, passes out at the slightest provocation, is as pale as marble, and has a nagging cough. Most likely the ethereal swooner is under-nourished, anemic, and chronically constipated, and has problems with "the curse."[18] It is taxing to imagine her taking two dance classes a day.

COMPETING WITH THE SYLPH

Every generation laughs at the old fashions, but follows religiously the new.
 —Henry David Thoreau

A glance at early photographs of dancers reveals not only how subtly our concept of beauty has crept up on us, but also that one doesn't have to be a sylph to portray one. Consider one of the favorite ballerinas of the 1840s, Fanny Cerrito, by comparing her engraved portrait with an actual photograph (figure 4). In the engraving she is floating in space like a wisp, her repose not initiated by a leap but by a gust of wind, perhaps only a slight draft. Suspended by the buoyancy of the air, she is not merely light, she is weightless.

In the photograph she is considerably weightier. To say she has an abundant bustline and sturdy legs would be downplaying at best. Frankly, one would hate to run into such a substantial frame in a dark studio; she appears as solid as the Chrysler Building and possibly as tough to lift off the ground. In all fairness, it must be noted that this photograph was taken toward the end of her career, when even her contemporaries viewed her as more than adorably plump, with a few critics going so far as to hint that she was still a marvelous dancer "in spite of her figure."[19]

But few will dispute that dancers were heavier back then; we need not traverse a century to see the insidious change, to realize that our eyes have been blurred by the deceit of art and fashion. Comparing the current generation of dancers with those of the more recent past, we note that while the physical demands have become greater, the trend is thinner and thinner, paralleling the society as a whole. Again, this is not to deny the dancer's need to be thin; it is a question of the working definition of thinness and of the standards by which the criteria are established.

The renowned principal ballerina Alexandra Danilova maintained an "ideal" dancing weight of approximately 112 pounds for her nearly five-foot-five-inch frame throughout a career which lasted for more than three decades. Yet one of her current students, considered to have an excellent ballet stature and of roughly the same height and bone structure as Mme. Danilova, dances at a weight of 91 pounds. In light of this, it is even more ironic to hear the young woman disparagingly comment on her lapses into relative obesity.

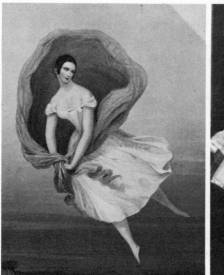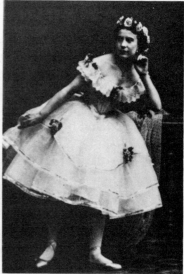

Figure 4: Fanny Cerrito as seen through the eyes of an engraver (left) and as seen through the eyes of a camera (right). In the former she is light on her feet; in the latter, she is considerably weightier (it appears that a well-placed jeté might precipitate a major landslide).

(Reproductions courtesy of the Dance Collection, The New York Public Library at Lincoln Center, Astor, Lenox, and Tilden Foundations)

"You should have seen me at 102," she told me. "I looked awful."

Paradoxically, when you consider the exceptional dancers in ballet, the guidelines for an "ideal" look have little, if any, meaning whatsoever. It doesn't take particularly astute vision to realize that such ballet dancers as Cynthia Gregory, Patricia McBride, Martine van Hamel, Gelsey Kirkland, Natalia Makarova, Suzanne Farrell, and Carla Fracci do not conform to any particular mold. And many might not consider Judith Jamison to have a "dancer's body" until, of course, they have seen her dance. What distinguishes these and other fine dancers from others far transcends height, weight, extension, and bustline. A technically competent dancer with the "right look" is one thing, but the special dancers are another breed entirely. They are unique, and the sum total of all the intangibles allows them to overcome virtually anything.

> A New York City ballet instructor observes: If you look at the dancers who're around today, or the great artists of the past, very few of them are physically perfect. They all have something wrong; either short arms, short legs, short torso, too big, too tall, wide ears, eyes crossed. There's always something wrong with them somewhere, but they learn to make it work for them. They move so well, and they're so coordinated, that you don't notice that maybe their arms are too short for their body . . . you never really see it.

> And Mme. Danilova puts it in these terms: "For dancing you have to have talent, and you have to have the look. If you don't have the look, then you have to have double talent. Because your talent makes people forget how you look."

Nonetheless, for the aspiring ballet dancer auditioning for the corps de ballet, there may be less latitude as far as individuality is concerned. The premium is on physicality, and often the expectations—either as they are demanded in fact or as they are perceived—might actually be ill suited to the business of dancing.

> [Some companies] are missing out on a lot of wonderful dancers because they're picking a body type, they're not necessarily picking a talented dancer. And this is where one has to be very, very careful. That you don't just get caught up on someone because of the way they look physically, rather than to take someone who really has a feel for dance, who after careful training and refinement, can maybe lengthen out that sort of square-looking body. It doesn't mean to say because that body isn't long and thin that it shouldn't dance.

The insight and benevolence of the dance instructor whom I quote was marred somewhat by the following addendum, an expression of an attitude which I find quite prevalent among young dancers, and one which is bothersome in its implications:

> But if your structure is short and thick—muscular thick— then it has to be *down to the bone*, and if you can get it down to the bone without being ill, fine. If you can't, then you've got to get out of it.

A seventeen-year-old girl comes to clinic weighing ninety-five pounds, convinced that something is wrong with her thyroid because she can't lose the "fat" from her muscular thighs. A fifteen-year-old girl who resembles a curtain rod is on a liquid protein regimen for weight control, under the supervision of a physician and with the consent and encouragement of her stage mother. A five-foot-three-inch tall ballet scholarship student, barely tipping the scale at one hundred pounds, wants advice on how to reduce to eighty-five pounds in two weeks for an audition.

Obviously it is easier for some people to conform to a given look than others. But the competition is always relative, usually needless, often futile, and perhaps self-destructive—be it the short, compact dancer competing with the long, thin one, or the long, thin one competing with the sylph. Preoccupation with weight, when the expectations are unrealistic, amounts to an ominous distortion.

Metabolic Illusion Versus Reality

THE DUPED DANCER

To preserve one's health by too strict a
regimen is in itself a tedious malady.
—François, duc de La Rochefoucauld

So convenient a thing it is to be a *reasonable creature* since it enables one to find or
make a reason for every thing one has a
mind to do.
—Benjamin Franklin

Often I espy unhealthy-looking patrons coming from or going
into health food stores. Not wishing to belittle these establish-
ments, I only want to point out that 1) "healthy foods" don't
necessarily have to be "health foods"; and 2) concern with eating
does not insure proper eating. Consumers may be victimized by
oddball diets, misleading product promotion, or outright fake
food cures. Sir William Osler noted that "the greater the
ignorance, the greater the dogmatism," and in the business of
nutrition, a little ignorance can go a long way. Dancers and other
athletes, often looking for something to give them an edge,
competitive or otherwise, are especially vulnerable to being
duped. Granted, compared to hard work and training, a nutritional magic wand would be an easy way out. A New York
physician analyzed this peculiar blind spot: "They [dancers] are
so involved in their bodies, and the minute changes that happen
to their bodies, that they are willing to listen to anything.
Anything that ranges from utter nonsense to sense, but they have
no standard of judgment. . . . It's their bodies and how they
perform; there's nothing else in their lives, and they know it.
And here you are—this sort of normal person interviewing
them—and how can they tell you about the fanaticism? I mean,
they're embarrassed."

Up to a point, and if one turns a cynical eye on nutritional
history, food fallacies may not have dire consequences and may
be appreciated simply for their own sake. For example, when
ordering a sandwich on whole wheat, I am mindful of a great

tradition. Hippocrates would no doubt have made the same choice, as he recommended unbolted wheat meal for its "salutary effect upon the bowels." The Greek wrestlers ate a coarse dark bread, and according to Pliny, the Romans subsisted on it in the days of their greatest glory. Nibbling on the crust, I recall that the Emperor Augustus did the same while bouncing about in his chariot seeking new worlds to conquer, as did Seneca (he stressed eating it in the standing position, however). For even more reassurance, I think back on Sylvester Graham, who promised his generation that they would all live to be a hundred if they ate brown bread. In brief, even if it's a rotten sandwich and the bread is stale, I can still feel pretty exhilarated about every mouthful.

On the other hand, if I happen to select white bread (drawing dirty, condescending glances and/or comments from ardently "health-conscious" eaters), I rationalize that it is vitamin fortified, that I probably have an adequate fiber content in my diet from other foods, that my digestive juices really get into gear with foods I find palatable, and, finally, that Sylvester Graham— despite the fact that he was famous enough to have a cracker named after him—wasn't really all that reliable. In addition to pushing brown bread with incredible zeal, he claimed that condiments caused the blues and led to insanity, tea produced delirium tremens, meat eating inflamed the "baser propensities," and both chicken pie and lewdness caused cholera.[20] To further dampen his credibility, Sylvester died at the age of fifty-seven.

"Too strict a regimen" and wholesale acceptance of food fads can lead to any number of pitfalls. Excerpts from an interview which I conducted with a young ballet student who is very concerned about eating "appropriately" in order to help her dancing as well as maintain her weight, are quite illustrative:

Dancer: I've tried everything. Like the pineapple diet. For two days I ate nothing but fresh pineapple.
Vincent: Why did you quit?
Dancer: Because it hurt my tongue [laughter]; and you're only

supposed to go on it for two days because after that you get
weak. And then I got really sick and had to see a doctor
because I was just eating vegetables [gastrointestinal com-
plaints].
Vincent: When did you do this?
Dancer: For the next four days after the pineapple . . . then I
got sick. Also I was just taking liquids on the weekends . . . I
figured it didn't matter if I was weak on the weekends, just as
long as I ate protein and stuff during the week [for classes].
Vincent: What kind of liquids?
Dancer: I'd have carrot juice, and maybe I'd eat a carrot, but
mostly juices; orange juice or something like that.
Vincent: All weekend?
Dancer: And coffee, tea, diet soda, and lots of water.
Vincent: [Specifying needlessly] Coffee with Sweet 'N Low . . .
Dancer: Oh, yeah.
Vincent: How did you feel?
Dancer: I felt very loose on Monday.
Vincent: How was your endurance?
Dancer: Well, I could never really tell the difference between
being weak from not eating and exhausted from not getting
enough sleep.

[The dancer revealed that at the time of her dietary indiscretions, she was working four nights a week—getting home at
about eleven P.M.—dancing four to six hours a day, and getting
up at six A.M. to do correspondence work for her high school
equivalency. After the pineapple/vegetable/liquid regimen
had met with less than positive results, the dancer embarked
on a low carbohydrate diet—occasionally "splurging" on a
grapefruit—for about three weeks.]
Vincent: But you're aware that you need carbohydrates for energy?
Dancer: Yeah, I found that out.
Vincent: How?
Dancer: Getting spaced-out all the time. I didn't have enough
energy. I know that I could pretty much eat what I want to,

three meals a day, basically fifteen hundred or maybe two thousand calories a day, and I might be five or seven pounds heavier than I am now, and maintain that without any problem.

Vincent: So you think that the weight you want to attain for ballet may be unnatural for you?

Dancer: It is.

Vincent: So why? Why do you go through all this business?

Dancer: Because I want to be good.

Food faddism may be financially costly, may cause the dancer to credit satisfaction and success to other things besides talent and hard work, and may also inhibit the development of optimum performing capabilities. Unnecessary measures need not be hazardous in themselves to be detrimental; taken to extremes, they may exclude healthful practices and be harmful indirectly. For instance, fatigue precipitated by inadequate nutritional reserves might make one more susceptible to a musculoskeletal injury, assuredly a more tangible problem than the loss of pep from which it resulted.

Faddist tendencies aside, emphasis on slimness in itself may result in miserable eating habits. One professional ballet dancer treated her dietary intake with characteristic abandon:

Vincent: What did you eat yesterday?

Dancer: I had a bowl of onion soup and some bread.

Vincent: All day?

Dancer: Yeah, and some coffee [laughter]. About three cups of coffee. But I'm going to start eating more.

Vincent: What did you eat the day before?

Dancer: I don't know; I don't think I ate. Oh, I had some yogurt.

Vincent: All day?

Dancer: Yes; and some coffee.

Vincent: With sugar?

Dancer: Sweet 'N Low.

It invariably boils down to misplaced priorities. The conscientious eater may be conscientious about everything except eating; never skimping on daily vitamins—sometimes in mega-doses—or supplements such as lecithin, dolomite, wheat germ, and the like, but somehow forgetting that energy is derived from food. The end result may be a suboptimal nutritional state with a vitamin-enriched urine (most vitamin excesses are rapidly excreted by the kidney, particularly the water-soluble B and C vitamins). The dancer quoted above was somewhat shocked to learn that her interviewer occasionally indulged in "regular" cola, as she was quite concerned about avoiding "junk" calories. Without question, purified sugars are much too large a compo-nent of the daily caloric intake of the average American (and have been implicated in the causation of conditions such as obesity, diabetes, and coronary artery disease), but in light of her own dietary regimen, perhaps a few "junk" calories would have been better than no calories at all.

Once priorities have been misplaced or an erroneous premise accepted, bad habits or fallacies may be perpetuated through *misattribution,* the attributing of a symptom to an incorrect cause. Take the dancer who lacks "pep" in her last class of the day. Perhaps she will blame hypoglycemia, or failure to take enough B vitamins, brewer's yeast, or Tiger's Milk. By some twisted reason of logic, the fact that she has had only a cup of coffee and some yogurt for sustenance while dancing for six hours will not be perceived as a likely, or even possible, cause. Another dancer may blame her inability to lose weight on a metabolic derange-ment or hypothyroidism, discounting late-night cookie binges or her insistence on taking several Energol tablets every day (vitamin E in the form of wheat germ oil, with sixty calories concentrated in every capsule). And a young dancer may misattribute the dancing prowess of a contemporary to her diet of popcorn, Tab, and liquid protein, overlooking superior talent, discipline, and training and failing to comprehend that the dancer performs well not because of her diet, but in spite of it.

Misattribution in part stems from a confusing aspect of medical science: many ailments, major and minor, are heralded by symptoms which are the same, or relatively nonspecific. Additionally, false symptoms (normal physiological conditions such as low spirits, tiredness, tension, mild insomnia, and the like) may be mistaken for real symptoms. And since much of our interpretation of symptoms has a psychological component, we cannot always trust our perceptions of our own experience. It might still be argued that if one feels better with a particular offbeat regimen or unorthodox dietary manipulation—whether owing to a placebo effect or to an unknown or unsubstantiated biochemical alteration—then the regimen has some positive worth; that is, provided the regimen is not directly harmful in itself, or indirectly so in fostering a concomitant neglect of overall good health. Dietary idiosyncrasies may be viewed benevolently as long as they aren't idiocies. An awareness of some basic physiology may help to demarcate the difference.

A LESSON IN ENERGY METABOLISM

Perhaps someone should hire a large public relations firm to spruce up the image of "fat," the victim of a pervasive smear campaign. In common usage, we tend to think of fat as synonymous with obesity. This imprecision (which I am guilty of in this book) not only simplifies, but implicitly distorts. Obesity, without question, may be detrimental to good health. Shorter life expectancy and higher incidence of disease states such as hypertension, heart disease, and diabetes have a recognized relationship to obesity, public awareness of which has no doubt contributed to our culture's craving for slimness. But the negative aspects of an overabundance of fat have overshadowed the physiological importance of normal amounts. That an ounce of fat should be viewed as a near abomination exemplifies the irrationality and blind hatred directed toward our own distortion. In essence, we have become dietary McCarthyites, with fat filling in for the Communists.

For the human being, fat is the principal storage form of energy, accounting for approximately 80 to 85 percent of body fuel stores in the average nonobese man. This is a practical arrangement, since lipid (the highbrow designation for fat) is stored with very little water. Glycogen (the storage form of carbohydrate) and protein, on the other hand, are present in the body in association with water (the ratio of water to protein and glycogen is in the neighborhood of three or four to one). Thus, if man's primary energy reservoirs were relegated to protein and glycogen, he would be so bogged down with excess obligatory water weight that something as basic as moving would be quite an accomplishment.[21]

Lipid synthesis and storage are, in fact, a prerequisite to survival in any species that depends on motility. Not surprisingly, fat storage is most prominent in migratory insects and birds, as well as in seeds, pollens, fruits, and nuts (the latter relying on passive mobility for propagation of the species). This contrasts with carbohydrate as the major energy form in most of the plant kingdom (which may be one of many reasons why plants don't creep off the windowsill at night or watermelons have never been observed flying). Through painstaking evolution, metabolic processes for man have been selected which result in fat storage during periods of plenty (after the backup emergency reserves of liver and muscle glycogen have been filled) and fat depletion during leaner times. Protein may be called upon to stoke the metabolic fire, but it is preferentially spared as fuel by the body so it can fulfill its numerous nonfuel functions (as enzyme, contractile, or structural protein). Energy, then, is obtained from fat stores (in the form of free fatty acids) or from carbohydrate (in the form of liver glycogen, muscle glycogen, or circulating blood glucose), the relative contribution of each source being variable and determined by nutritional status and the amount (duration and intensity) of activity.

For intensive work, the glycogen stored in muscle is the most efficient energy source (we might view all-out physical activity as an "emergency" situation in Nature's eyes, since the energy burst required of a sprinter is not much different from the fuel needed by a primitive man being pursued by a fleet and hungry animal). Although glycogen is used preferentially with high intensity activity even in the presence of fatty acids and glucose, its use is restricted because of its limited supply. The Bluebird Variation from *The Sleeping Beauty,* for example, one of the most intense and demanding pieces in the classical repertory, only lasts about forty-five seconds. One would strain to imagine work of this speed and intensity persisting for another minute nonstop, let alone fifteen or twenty. Even the best-trained physical specimen can only go so far; at some point, the dancer's complexion might change to the color of his costume, he would be too pooped to execute another brisé volé. Depletion of muscle glycogen stores is associated with exhaustion.

Obviously, and of necessity, effort of this intensity for extended periods of time is not required in the day-to-day working or performing of the dancer or other athletes. Glycogen stores are somewhat protected by intermittent exercise, short periods of rest, or work of a lower intensity, which allows other fuels to assume more of the burden. In the resting state, muscles depend almost entirely on the oxidation of fatty acids. With exercise of low intensity, glucose becomes increasingly a more important source of energy. Free fatty acid use again predominates with prolonged mild exercise (after four hours); it is estimated that the relative contribution of fat becomes twice that of carbohydrate.[22] As exercise continues, amino acids—the basic components of protein—may be drafted into picking up some of the slack and aiding as a source of fuel (after first being converted into glucose). Obviously, optimum nutritional status for activity depends on much more than glycogen. Due credit should be given to fatty acids and glucose for getting one through several hours' worth of dancing.

FUEL MANAGEMENT AND TRANSFORMATION

Since the maintenance of a blood glucose level within certain limits is of high priority to the body (the major consumer of glucose is the brain, using roughly a fifth of the body's calories at rest), fine hormonal regulation is crucial, and the hormone insulin plays a major role (figure 5). Cells in the pancreas (called beta cells) constantly monitor blood sugar levels and release insulin accordingly. A slight rise in sugar levels, such as after a meal, augments insulin production. Relatively high levels of this hormone "open up" the body cells for the storage of fuel, removing the excess sugar (and other nutrients) from the bloodstream to bring the levels back to normal. In hungry states or with exercise—when glucose supplies in the circulating pool begin to dwindle—low levels of insulin initiate mobilization of fuels from storage, again to keep the glucose levels within a desirable range.[23]

If insulin is the principal fuel "coordinator," the major energy "transformer" in the body is the liver (figure 6), normally the sole site of production and release of glucose into the bloodstream (muscles lack the capability to convert glycogen into glucose for release into the blood, so muscle carbohydrate stores in one area are of little use for muscles elsewhere in the body). The liver can provide glucose in two ways: 1) from the breakdown of its own glycogen stores (a process called *glycogenolysis*); or 2) the production of glusoce *de novo* from glycerol, lactate, pyruvate, and certain amino aicds (a process called *gluconeogenesis*). Simply then, the fed state is characterized by high levels of insulin which instigate storage by the liver (a cessation of new glucose production and a replenishment of glycogen stores). The fasting state (and exercise), with low insulin levels, puts the transformer back into gear, breaking down its stores and increasing uptake of raw materials to function as the glucose distributor for the body.With exercise, the output of glucose from the liver may increase by more than two- or three-fold (for work of short duration, the increase is primarily an augmentation of glycogen breakdown, but there is a greater reliance on gluconeogenesis as exercise continues).

Because of the fine regulation and the adaptations made to meet the increased energy demands, the blood sugar levels change little in mild to moderate exercise, may increase somewhat with more severe exercise (attributed to the increased glucose production by the liver), and may decrease somewhat

Figure 5: Simplified schematic representation of regulation of blood sugar level by insulin via its effects on glucose production by the liver and mobilization of free fatty acids and amino acids

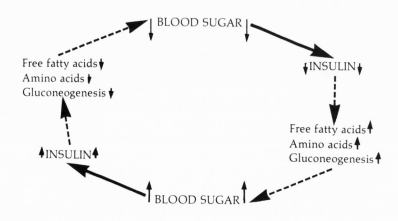

Figure 6: Schematic Representation: Derivation of Fuel Sources for Working Muscles

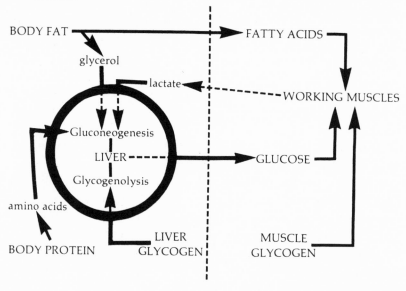

after extended exercise, though usually not to significantly low levels. Nonetheless, if liver glycogen stores are low (from prolonged exercise or low carbohydrate intake) and depleted fat stores restrict the availability of free fatty acids for energy needs, the liver may not be able to keep up with the glucose supplies demanded by exercise, and symptoms may result from significantly low blood sugar levels (hypoglycemia).[24]

HYPOGLYCEMIA: TAKING THE RAP

So let us backtrack to the ballet dancer who feels lousy at four o'clock every day and prefers to think that she suffers from a disease beyond her control (hypoglycemia) rather than to associate her fatigue with an overall poor nutritional status. Energy and vitality are commonly linked to blood sugar levels, and so lack of pep, fatigue, feeling down, or a poor performance all may be blamed on "hypoglycemia," which apparently has become the trendy, catchall explanation for a hodgepodge of vague, nonspecific symptoms experienced while dancing or in daily life (a fact well recognized and exploited by certain food gurus and nutritional supplement promoters). Granted, various disease states do exist in which hypoglycemia may eventuate, accompanied by symptoms such as fatigue, spasms, sweating, palpitations, and numbness. But low levels of blood sugar may normally occur after meals—when metabolism shifts from the fed to the fasting state—without any symptoms (in one study, 23 percent of normal control subjects showed glucose levels below 50 during glucose tolerance testing).[25]

An endocrinologist who deals extensively with dancers has frequently found "lowish" blood sugar levels in dancer patients, as well as in other young, very thin women. Patients with complaints of "hypoglycemia" often report disappearance of the symptoms when placed on an adequate diet (and not necessarily a high-protein, low-carbohydrate "hypoglycemia" diet). This observation isn't in the least surprising. Quoting the physician: "[The symptoms in these instances] are the result of terrible eating habits—call it whatever you want—but it's not a 'disease' and I think it happens constantly among dancers. The main causes are just poor diet, stress, and the fact that these people are underweight. People have to eat well to feel normal, and women are more sensitive to their diets than men."

To adequately diagnose a hypoglycemic condition, a physician should demonstrate that symptoms occur simultaneously with a nadir in blood glucose levels (some of the symptoms, such as sweating and palpitations, are the result of adaptive mechanisms, "stress" responses to low sugar levels intended to stimulate glucose output by the liver). The diagnosis, then, depends on two variables: the determination of an "abnormally" low blood glucose level and the association of symptoms with this level. Obviously, the first prerequisite requires some standard of what the normal range of blood sugar values is to begin with, and this is where the complexion of the medical profession was fairly recently found to be blemished.

The normal range for fasting blood glucose is generally accepted to be within 60 and 100 (milligrams glucose per 100 milliliters blood). It did not come to light until 1974, however, that the standard had been derived from control data from men and overweight women, but not from normal women. It was then demonstrated that for normal women, blood sugar levels do not necessarily stabilize at levels comparable to those for men;[26] in fact, they may occasionally dip to below 35mg/100ml without any symptoms. Reasons postulated for this discrepancy include the smaller muscular compartment for women and the influence of female sex hormones in modulating tissue uptake and utilization of glucose. Regardless of the explanation, erroneous standards for hypoglycemia in the past have undoubtedly contributed to the overestimation of the prevalence of this condition by physicians, as well as to the rampant popular urge to claim oneself its victim. Recent medical journal articles have emphasized the importance of distinguishing actual "chemical hypoglycemia" (which is treated by a low-carbohydrate, high-protein regimen and multiple meals) from the misattributed variety, termed "clinical pseudohypoglycemia" or "nonhypoglycemia."[27]

The main pitfall of any kind of misattribution is that the incorrect explanation may preclude the exploration of alternative explanations, and hence prevent appropriate intervention and correction of the problem. In the more specific case of pseudohypoglycemia in the dancer, "treatment" may conceivably make matters worse. Consider the hypothetical case of the "very thin" dancer who pursues a rigorous work schedule despite sparse fat stores and a suboptimal intake of carbohydrates. She experiences "lack of pep" in the afternoon and concludes that she is a "hypoglycemic" (as we have seen, if her liver can't keep up with the glucose demands, a physiologic hypoglycemic state with symptoms may in fact arise). Mistaking pseudohypoglycemia for chemical hypoglycemia, she places herself on a high-protein, low-carbohydrate diet. Thus, a condition that may have been initiated by an insufficient amount of carbohydrate (and generally poor nutritional status) is "remedied" by cutting back on carbohydrate even further. With continuance or exacerbation of the symptoms, a vicious nutritional cycle begins, making the dancer susceptible to further misattribution ("If it isn't hypoglycemia, it must be vitamin B deficiency, not enough brewer's yeast, etc.").

PIGGING-OUT

The thing I've noticed most of all is that
they [dancers] eat in excess; it's either
one or the other. Instead of cutting down
their food generally if they're trying to
lose weight, they just cut everything out.
And then they go from one extreme to
the other; they're starving one day and
they're gorging the next day.
    —Ballet Instructor, New York City

Dietary willpower comes easily to few of us, but nondancers rarely, if ever, have to submit to the degree of dietary denial and discipline that is for some dancers a matter of course. Yet dancers' eating patterns, particularly female dancers', often do not stay on an even keel. After carbohydrate denial, a number of dancers occasionally submit to a binge, succumbing to the likes of chocolate bars (Tobler Mocha), chocolate chip cookies (Entennman's), and ice cream (Häagen-Dazs rum raisin). To use the vernacular, "pigging-out" appears to be a conspicuous facet of the dance subculture.

Perhaps a definition of terms is needed, as one person's dessert might be another's pig-out. There is a considerable range between such a dietary indiscretion as à la mode with one's cake and a condition known as bulimia, compulsive eating of an extreme degree, usually followed by vomiting. Because of this subjective variability, I routinely asked ballet students to specify their "best" or "biggest" pig-outs. Representative samples included:

—A full dinner, followed by ice cream and one-third of a cheesecake;

—Bagel and cream cheese, a pint of ice cream, licorice candy, several cookies, a chocolate bar;

—Two pints of ice cream and a piece of baklava (followed by Ex-Lax);

—A piece of pizza, half a blueberry cheesecake, half a package of Vienna ladyfingers, half a bar of halvah, and a toasted English muffin (with butter).

Now, as legend has it, the Greek Olympic wrestling champion, Milo of Croton, once carried a four-year-old bull around an athletic stadium, killed it with a single blow, and ate it in one day. But whether or not this historical pig-out is exaggerated, we must keep in mind that Milo was big, bad, and mean. The weight range of the dancers whose indulgences I cite is between 100 and 125 pounds, certainly not in the wrestler's weight division.

For young dancers, pigging-out may be a social occasion—another example of the food-oriented direction that the cloistered milieu can take. In the words of a fledgling ballet company member, describing the antics of her cohorts residing in a woman's residence hall: "Everybody gets together and plans a day when they're going to buy everything they like to eat—all kinds of junk—and just eat and eat and eat it all. More or less it's just a party, but for us it's a pig-out, because we aren't supposed to do it."

The aftermath of the pig-out may be feelings of shame, guilt, anger, resignation, or depression; but whatever the reaction, amends can be made by subsequently stepping up dieting measures or—what is sometimes seen as more convenient and immediate expiation—self-induced vomiting or a bout of laxatives. Various factors might be responsible for this rebound eating, including the general preoccupation with food and any of a variety of psychological states (frustration, boredom, the blues). Interestingly enough, in my experience dancers who follow sensible diets not only tend to binge less frequently, but also consume considerably less when they do cheat. Perhaps, then, physiological factors are operating as well.

Researchers studying the extreme starvation of anorexia nervosa have noted that the severe carbohydrate restriction of these patients results in an abnormal insulin response to carbohydrate ingestion (high levels of insulin are sustained for longer periods than would be expected). It has been suggested that in these cases the abnormal response triggered by a small amount of carbohydrates leads to a compelling need to continue eating carbohydrates.[28] In other words, perhaps abstinence from carbohydrates can lead to a greater carbohydrate dependency and cravings that precipitate a binge.

We might speculate on the possibility of a similar mechanism's contributing to pigging-out among dancers who routinely maintain severe carbohydrate restriction. If this is the case, carbohydrate denial may backfire in two ways: not only will dancing efficiency be jeopardized, but dieting efforts may be hampered by the clash of willpower against physiological needs.

ADAPTATIONS, THE UNSEEN VARIABLE

We may wonder how some dancers manage to subsist on relatively meager food intakes, sometimes compounding the situation by dieting. Not surprisingly, we find that physiological adaptations are at work, enabling the body to get the most (and the best) mileage per calorie.

Athletic training in itself makes one a more efficient energy machine. Compare a principal ballerina doing a series of combinations across a studio floor with a less trained and less skilled counterpart (they may both be the same height, weight, and age, have the exact body type, or even be identical twins, if you will). The latter dancer, not as smooth or as proficient at execution as the former, must exert more effort in accomplishing the steps and maintaining balance; she is working harder and using more energy (burning more calories) than the accomplished dancer. But to begin with, since the number of calories required by an individual depends on the amount of body tissue needed to be maintained, a 95-pound female dancer will obviously be able to get by on fewer calories than a 170-pound male. Thus, not only may a dancer require relatively few calories because of diminutive size, but skill may minimize the energy expenditure entailed by physical activity.

Another factor is that when nutritional intake is inadequate, the body allows the greatest possible leeway through the establishment of its priorities. We know that the body makes efforts to conserve its protein, but when this is no longer possible, low levels of insulin signal the breakdown of protein and its mobilizatiion as fuel. But exercise counteracts this effect; muscle contraction inhibits protein breakdown and stimulates protein synthesis—the long-term effect of repeated muscular work being muscle buildup (hypertrophy), not wasting. So for the dancer who is not eating well, if protein breakdown is to occur, it will occur preferentially from the muscles that are *not* being worked, which is why dancers may be quite bony in the chest and arms and still maintain well-delineated, hypertrophied leg musculature.

Aside from the "local" sparing of certain tissues in nutritional hard times, the body in its entirety makes adaptations. Classic studies of prolonged caloric restriction have shown that fasting subjects have a decrease in metabolic rate, exhibit a voluntary decrease in the amount of physical activity undertaken, and derive a greater percentage of energy from available fat depots (conserving body protein and water). The body establishes priorities which enable it to function as well as possible under adverse conditions, slowing down its furnace and becoming quite miserly in order to get the most out of the available energy. It seems likely that some dancers perpetrate their own energy crisis in the name of "the look," forcing the body to compensate and pick up the slack. Ultimately, the result may be a suboptimal diet, suboptimal energy reserves, and difficulty in climbing out of this self-excavated metabolic rut.

The War with Water and Salt

Talk to a dancer about her weight and you are apt to hear the phrase, "I retain water." Alas, a loaded statement. It seems almost a heartbreaking confession, a profound admission of a preordained curse or scandal.

"I am a deviant. Didn't you know? *I retain water.* No pity, please. Stoically shall I accept my fate, against all odds make special efforts and allowances to contend with my handicap. In the end, my talent shall reign supreme!"

Such a dramatic conception is not actually the case. Water retention is not a special disease, it is a normal phenomenon. In the words of a female endocrinologist: "Every woman retains fluid. I retain fluid. I can wake up in the morning and I can have puffy eyes. But it doesn't matter to me. I'm not on stage and I'm not looking in a mirror all day long."

Cyclical variations in water weight, then, which many women experience and accept as a matter of course, often becomes an intolerable situation for dancers.

Five pounds of water may not be much for someone weighing 150 pounds, but for a 95-pound dancer, it's more than 5 percent of her total body weight. She can see it in the mirror and she can feel it. And then there are the constant reminders, such as having difficulty in hooking a costume or imagining a louder grunt from the male partner doing the lifting. Most importantly, the water weight unfortunately assumes the dimensions of a lost skirmish in the war against fat. In the light of an innocently disguised but vindictive "Put on some weight?" fat and water become virtually indistinguishable, and the immediate response is the resolve to intensify dieting efforts. This works both ways, of course, for a compliment on looking "good" is a substantial morale booster, even if a diuretic is responsible. In either case, the actual amount of body fat may not have changed a fraction of an iota; only perceptions have altered, in what amounts to a self-involved game.

Although the difference in weight caused by water retention may be noticeable and distressing, the dancer's reaction to it is often completely out of proportion. An orthopedist relates an example of this hypersensitivity, giving insight as well into some of the special difficulties a physician may encounter in a practice dealing with dancers. In his practice, the orthopedist frequently prescribes the anti-inflammatory agent Butazolidin (phenylbutazone) for soft tissue injuries. One of the side effects of this medication is salt retention (and hence water retention), which completely resolves upon cessation of the drug but is nonetheless often unacceptable for the physician's dancer patients. At the mention of the drug, "right away they say 'that puts on weight.' Right away. They know it causes water retention, and they want to know if they can take a diuretic with it, or they won't take it unless you give them a diuretic with it. You have to explain to them that you're treating their present condition in time, and that as soon as the inflammatory stage is over, they discontinue the medication and the water will leave them."

Getting them to use the drug may, reports the physician, require considerable coaxing and compromising. Similarly, a number of dancers will not employ oral contraceptives precisely because of their water-retaining characteristics.

Water retention is a problem healthy men never have to deal with, since the fluid excess primarily results from the salt-retaining properties of the female hormone estrogen. During the premenstrual period (when estrogen levels are relatively highest), normal women show a slight gain of weight (in one study, 30 percent of women gained three or more pounds).[29] The weight gain may occasionally be greater and may be accompanied by puffiness of the face and eyes and swelling of the feet or ankles. Toward the beginning of the period, or sometimes immediately after its cessation, increased urination causes rapid disappearance of the surplus reservoir. Of course, hormonal factors are only one variable in water balance, so let us step back for a broader overview in order to examine the dancer's dealings with matters liquid.

A LESSON IN WATER BALANCE

The ground rules for water balance are straightforward. The losses incurred through urine, feces, and sweating (as well as that lost by diffusion through the skin and the water vapor contained in exhaled air) must not exceed the amount which is supplied through intake of fluids, liquid content of foods, and the smaller quantity produced by the body during metabolism of food for energy. It is not possible for man to adapt, or be physically trained, to tolerate water intake lower than daily losses.

Under any circumstances dehydration severely compromises the body's ability to function in a variety of ways—and dancing on top of it can only make matters worse. In part, a dancer's endurance is limited by the capacity of the circulatory system to provide oxygen and nutrients to the working muscles. But the increased body heat produced by exercise also requires greater blood flow to the skin to dissipate heat by vaporizing sweat. Of course, there is a limited amount of blood for all these jobs (the blood volume of a 100-pound ballet dancer may be estimated at less than 3½ quarts). The more sweating, the greater the amount of body fluids lost, and the less blood there is to go around. Spreading oneself (or one's fluids) too thinly may impair performance and efficiency in early stages; carried to an extreme, it results in collapse (in some cases fatal).

The average adult water loss is in the neighborhood of 2 liters (slightly more than two quarts) per day; the daily average water allowance for adults is thus often quoted as 2.5 liters. For the individual of average activity, water intake and losses balance very closely, and daily weight fluctuations related to water are usually less than 1 percent of body weight. The athlete, on the other hand, may regularly incur a short-term negative water balance of 2 to 3 percent of body weight during daily exercise, and may in some cases reach the critical 5 percent dehydration level. The capabilities for sweat loss are awesome; an individual exercising vigorously in a hot environment can lose as much as eight pounds of water weight as sweat in a period of an hour.[30] Water intake must correspond to the increased water loss; free access to fluids is imperative to minimize dehydration and reduce the threat of overheating. Usually the sensation of thirst will govern replenishment over a twenty-four-hour period (more than five pounds may be regained in a few hours after eating and drinking), although in some instances, with episodes of continued bouts of dehydration, thirst may be inadequate to insure sufficient intake.

There are much more subtle mechanisms operating to maintain water (and salt) balance besides the sensations of thirst and hunger. For example, with training and heat acclimation, the concentration of a dancer's sweat becomes more diluted—an adaptation of the body to diminish salt loss. Although the sweat glands produce this modification, the principal responsibility for regulating water and salt balance is relegated to the kidneys. Both the amount of fluid excreted as urine and the salt concentration in the fluid are variable. In response to heavy sweating and periods of dehydration, the kidneys adjust accordingly, reducing the excretion of both salt and water.

Two hormones primarily mediate these modifications by the kidney. Antidiuretic hormone (ADH) is released by the pituitary gland under the control of a part of the brain called the hypothalamus. The mechanism is as follows: receptors in the hypothalamus detect changes in concentration of the blood; with water deprivation (or a relative loss of water from excessive sweating), more of the hormone is released into the bloodstream, causing the kidney to excrete less water in the urine. The second hormone, aldosterone, is secreted by the adrenal gland in greater amounts when the circulating blood volume is decreased (such as in a state of salt deficiency and dehydration). Aldosterone acts on the renal tubules, enhancing the body's reabsorption of sodium and chloride (potassium and hydrogen are lost in the process). The enhanced salt retention will secondarily lead to greater water retention.

DANCERS AND DEHYDRATION

If one didn't know any better, one might get the impression that

certain dancers are intentionally bent on dehydrating themselves. The loss of body water is greatest in hot, humid
conditions, because higher temperatures require more cooling
and increased humidity decreases the ease with which the body
moisture evaporates. If environmental conditions aren't bad
enough, dancers often create their own personal "hothouse"
with rubber suits or layer upon layer of warm-up clothes. Worse
yet, some will pursue sweat sessions while simultaneously
restricting intake of water and salt, an outlandishly stupid and
dangerous practice.

A common notion is that one isn't working hard unless sweat
is dripping. But since dripping sweat does not conduct the body's
heat by vaporizing, it does not cool effectively. Hence, a puddle
of water at one's feet represents a sacrifice of body fluids with
very little cooling to show for it. Not that dripping sweat can be
avoided; but if one is a "heavy sweater," starting to drip might
serve as a signal to remove a layer of warmings or, at the very
least, to be sure to take an appropriate amount of water to
compensate for increased losses.

Diuretics (water pills) enhance the excretion of body water,
and hence potentially may precipitate or compound dehydration. Nevertheless, individual athletes of all varieties—wrestlers,
boxers, jockeys, lightweight crew—still persist in employing
dehydration techniques to "make weight," and in my experience, dancers are no exception. Diuretics are not indicated
unless prescribed by a doctor, in which case they should be used
gingerly (a hard-working dancer might be wise to be somewhat
stoical about cyclical water retention). Physicians are sometimes
inclined to dispense diuretics against their better judgment in an
effort to appease stubborn and demanding patients. Also, a
conniving patient may purposely exaggerate the extent of water
retention in an effort to present a stronger argument for
unnecessary medication.

Ironically, in their concerted efforts to rid themselves of water,
dancers may actually be perpetrating the opposite condition, the
subsequent (temporary) accumulation of even more water. This

slap in the face by Mother Nature might occur under two similar conditions. I have already mentioned that the kidney responds to a dehydrated state or salt deficit by increasing the production of the hormone aldosterone, thereby promoting sodium retention. Researchers have shown that when water is consumed freely during repeated workouts in the heat, the body actually retains salt (and thus water) to an increased extent.[31] In other words, repeated bouts of dehydration may eventuate in the body's storing water in excess of the sweat loss. Thus, bundling up like an Eskimo and inducing dehydration may result in greater rehydration after one's thirst has been appeased (a phenomenon which I refer to as "Nanook's Revenge").

Similarly, it appears that people accustomed to low salt intakes may not excrete a heavy salt load effectively (possibly also due to higher aldosterone levels). For instance, if a dancer who normally shuns sodium eats a salty pastrami sandwich for dinner, she may find herself more "blown up" than usual the next morning (an acute case of the "Post-Pastrami Puffs").

WATER AND DIETING

For dieters, the contribution of water to the total amount of weight loss or gain can be frustrating and deceiving. Most of the total body weight is water—roughly 60 percent for the average man and closer to 50 percent for the average woman. The difference reflects the fact that fatty tissue contains only about 20 percent water, whereas muscle is nearly 75 percent; thus, the more muscular the individual, the greater the total percentage of body water. Generally, women have a higher fat content than men, but this may not be true in the lean, small-busted dancer with narrow hips, who in all likelihood may contain even more water per pound than most males.

Knowing that such a high percentage of body weight is water, one may easily appreciate that rapid weight fluctuations are always the result of fluid shifts and have nothing to do with the fate of fat. Any dieter tends to lose weight more quickly the first week or two of dieting, and much of this initial loss is water (in a recent study, 66 percent of the weight lost in the early phases of a diet was water).[32] Although the mechanism is incompletely understood, early or semi-starvation is characterized by increased sodium concentration in the urine and by reduction in the concentrating ability of the kidneys, which would account for greater water losses. Additionally, as I have mentioned previously, protein and glycogen are incorporated into the body tissue along with water. Thus, as glycogen stores are depleted in fasting or carbohydrate deprivation, there is an obligatory water loss (perhaps 600–800ml). Water losses are less of a factor in the later stages of a diet; in fact, water retention may even account for a gain in weight despite ongoing net losses of fat and protein.

The type of diet upon which one embarks also affects the amount of weight loss attributable to water. A comparison of low carbohydrate diets with mixed diets (both with the same number of calories) reveals that differences in weight loss are almost entirely attributable to the higher rate of water loss in the low carbohydrate regimens.[33] Semi-starvation and severe carbohydrate restriction are also difficult to sustain and are not satisfactory approaches from the standpoint of meeting a dancer's energy needs. The most productive loss of fat results from a steady restriction of caloric intake and/or increased energy expenditure over the long haul. In general, the quality of weight loss is likely to be the highest (a high percentage of fat being metabolized rather than increased water and protein losses) when the rate of loss is the slowest.

Because the percentage of water loss is highest in the beginning stages of dieting and the amount of water loss can be accentuated and prolonged in dieters either on low carbohydrate diets or simply fasting, we can understand why so many are thwarted in dieting efforts. In the beginning, when there is wholehearted conviction and dedication to the cause of dietary denial, weight loss according to the scale is apt to be the greatest and psychologically most gratifying. As the resolve weakens with the passing days, so does the positive feedback. A slip-up, such as succumbing to forbidden or salty foods, causes increased fluid retention and thus discouragement from the scale. With so many factors coming into play—recurrent bouts of dehydration from sweating, normal physiological fluid shifts from hormonal changes, unpredictability of eating behavior, and the variability with which water is lost in various types (as well as phases) of dietary regimens—it is no wonder that one cannot always trust one's eyes when looking a scale squarely in the face, or even when gazing at the mirrored wall.

ELECTROLYTES AND HYPOKALEMIA

Though salt loss always accompanies sweating, the concentration of salt in sweat is only one-third to one-half that of the blood. Therefore, relatively more water than salt is lost through perspiration, so the need for promptly replacing water is greater and more immediate than the demand for salt. Salt pills or special salt solutions are not necessary at the studio; a plain water fountain will suffice, provided the diet is adequate in replacing the salt losses at mealtimes. Sodium and chloride are the principal mineral elements in sweat; potassium and magnesium are lost in smaller amounts. Since these and other elements have the property of carrying an electrical charge when dissolved in solution (as ions), they are commonly referred to as electrolytes.

Certainly excessive sweating, in combination with poor or restricted dietary intake of salt and minerals, may result in a deficiency state, such as low sodium levels (hyponatremia), hand in hand with dehydration. Despite the body's compensatory salt-sparing mechanisms (such as decreased excretion of sodium in both sweat and urine during heat acclimation), dietary means dominate in the maintenance of water and electrolyte balance. Salt deficiency in a healthy individual can always be avoided by sensible eating and drinking; far from being an occupational hazard of the dance, it results from neglect. Sometimes more than neglect may be involved, however, which a consideration of potassium will reveal.

Potassium serves numerous important functions in the body: it is involved in energy-consuming reactions and the formation of high energy compounds; it aids in the synthesis of glucose and glycogen; and its relative concentration (on the inside as compared to the outside of muscle cells) is instrumental in the normal functioning of muscles. The principal symptom of low potassium (hypokalemia) is marked fatigue, primarily due to the role of the ion in muscular contraction. A person may experience weakness or numbness, or in severe instances, partial or even complete paralysis (usually in the extremities). Other possible ramifications of hypokalemia include electrocardiogram changes, irregular heart rhythms (potentially fatal), and damage to the kidneys.

Because potassium is widely distributed in foods such as oranges, grapefruit, bananas, beef, and fish; and since the body is particularly efficient in controlling normal levels of this electrolyte, potassium deficiency is highly unlikely to develop under normal circumstances. Disturbingly, the problem can nonetheless occur in dancers as the sequela of self-inflicted abnormal circumstances. Commonly, dancers who know something of hypokalemia—from firsthand experience or word of mouth—assume the condition to be the unavoidable result of heavy sweating. This is hardly the case.

As I have mentioned, a reasonable diet should be adequate to restore electrolyte balance in spite of excessive sweating. But in fact, potassium is not lost through perspiration to a large extent anyway. The concentration of sodium in sweat is roughly ten times that of potassium; nine pounds of sweat contain an estimated 6 to 8 percent of the body's sodium and chloride, but less than 1 percent of the body's potassium and magnesium.[34]

Then how can potassium deficiency come about? Aside from disease states (such as kidney disorders or diseases producing steriod hormones or requiring them for treatment), there are only two ways in which excessive potassium can be lost: 1) by rapid, heavy, or prolonged diuresis (urination); or 2) through the gastrointestinal tract (by vomiting or excessive diarrhea). Here is where electrolyte disturbances may be the direct consequence of self-abusive practices (figure 7).[35]

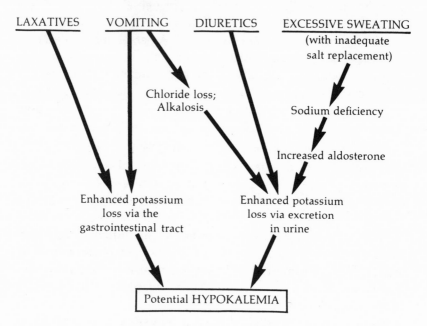

Figure 7: Mechanisms of Increased Potassium Loss

The excessive diarrhea prompted by the habitual overuse of laxatives, as well as the increased urination induced by diuretics (especially the thiazide types, furosimide, and ethacrynic aicd), may substantially enhance potassium wastage (patients treated with potassium-losing diuretics for high blood pressure are either given potassium supplements or advised to ingest potassium-rich foods, and their potassium levels are intermittently monitored). Continual and repeated vomiting results in a loss not only of ingested potassium-containing foods, but also of the acid contents of the stomach (gastric juices). Prolonged, unreplaced losses of body acid (and accompanying chloride ions) may lead to the pH of the body becoming more alkaline, prompting the kidney to compensate by excreting more base (bicarbonate) in the urine. But along with the bicarbonate (and due to the losses of chloride), the amount of potassium in the urine increases also. Thus, self-induced vomiting may account for greater potassium wastage through both the urinary and the gastrointestinal routes.

The specific problem of potassium deficiency is difficult to isolate from the general one of salt and water imbalance. For example, although perspiration may not be a major medium for potassium loss, the loss of sodium in sweat may have an indirect effect. Recall that a state of low sodium with dehydration will induce greater retention of sodium by the kidney via the hormone aldosterone. The mechanism involves a "trade-off" of electrolytes; sodium is kept preferentially at the expense of a greater loss of potassium in the urine. In this manner, excessive and unreplaced sodium losses may contribute to additional potassium wastage as the body attempts to remedy the deficit.

Since approximately 98 percent of the body's potassium resides within the cells, the amount in the blood—be it low, normal, or high—may not necessarily reflect the body's potassium status. The kidneys happen to be more responsive to high blood levels of potassium than to low ones, which is another manner in which subtle losses may occur. As potassium is closely related to stored glycogen, the breakdown of glycogen for energy may produce a temporary elevation of blood potassium levels, prompting the kidneys to excrete some of this excess in the urine. In this way, bringing the blood level back to normal in effect contributes to a gradual depletion of the total body stores, even though the blood level gives no indication of this. Potassium loss is a slow, insidious process.

A New York City physician described a teenage dancer patient who was so chronically deficient in potassium that she experienced paralysis in her feet and lower legs and compromised kidney function. Obviously this deficiency did not occur overnight, and the patient fervently denied any "wrongdoing" on her part. Patients often fail to admit to laxative or diuretic abuse, or to self-induced vomiting, which can greatly hamper a physician's clinical assessment. Certainly, in matters such as these, experienced physicians have a high index of suspicion. As one stated: "I am convinced that many of the dancers [with electrolyte imbalances] who have told me things have just not told me the whole story. You may not always know what people do to themselves, because they lie to you constantly."

It is impossible to assess the extent of hypokalemia in the dance world or to determine whether relative deficiencies might be related to some of the common complaints of dancers, such as weakness and fatigue. But in a healthy person subsisting on a reasonable diet, the condition should not occur. Nor, under normal circumstances, should potassium supplements be required for an individual (in fact, potassium supplements may be the cause of stomach upsets—besides, the liquid stuff tastes terrible). I am reminded of a dancer on voluntary water and salt restriction (and possibly laxative abuse), who sneakily attempted to second-guess physiology by self-prescribing over-the-counter potassium replacements. Although she avoided hypokalemia (her potassium levels were actually too high), she was foiled nonetheless, collapsing immediately after a performance because of dehydration and hyponatremia. At some point, foolishness will always tax the body beyond its gracious benevolence.

DIGRESSION: ON LEG WARMERS

In the summer of 1924, a group of three singers, a conductor, and four dancers—under the name of the Soviet State Dancers—took leave from the Maryinsky Theatre for a summer vacation period. State-sanctioned permission to cross the Baltic ultimately meant defection for the organizer of the tour, a baritone in the Maryinsky Opera Company named Vladimir Dimitriev, and the troupe of dancers, which included George Balanchine, Tamara Geva, Alexandra Danilova, and Nicholas Efimov.

After several lean and hungry years in revolutionary Russia, the troupe literally gorged on the abundance of food that was available for the two-and-a-half days of the Baltic crossing, and at least as far as Alexandra Danilova was concerned, this was only the beginning. She described to me with relish the whipped cream and other culinary delights in which she indulged in Berlin, to the extent that in three months she had reached 130 pounds (a surplus of about 18 pounds).

At Danilova's first rehearsal with the Diaghilev Company in Paris, the famous dancer Anton Dolin, faced with the prospect of having to partner such an abundant package, remarked to her: "You know what? I am not a piano mover, I am a dancer." It was the great impresario himself who presented Danilova with the ultimatum. Either she would lose weight, or Diaghilev would give her nothing to dance. At age twenty, Danilova—who throughout her career at the Maryinsky had never been admonished about her weight—learned firsthand the metabolic facts of life of the dance world.

Her reaction was to go immediately to a well-stocked pharmacy on the Champs Élysées, where she procured an unknown variety of diet pills (Madame Danilova only remembers that the packaging had "before" and "after" figures on it, one odiously fat and the other impressively thin). Convinced that the medication was the easy remedy to her problem, she raced back to her hotel with her purchase to initiate her diet. In her eagerness and desperation, Danilova fell victim to an all-too-common flaw in logic. The package directions called for one pill, one or two times a day. The ballerina said to herself, "One pill? Why one? I take five pills!"—a course of action which she followed, and which shortly thereafter resulted in her passing out.

Her next recollection was of Balanchine shaking her and inquiring about what had happened to his sick, trembling, and crying companion—and then condemning her for being so stupid as to resort to taking the pills. He offered instead some of his own dietary advice, which, as Danilova recalls, included eating meat and avoiding ice cream and other sweets. He also recommended that she take two daily lessons and "get warm clothes." The purpose was to make her perspire, for as Danilova so wonderfully states with her Russian inflection, perspiration "to get all grease out" was of high priority in her weight-reducing regimen.

Danilova related how she cut the sleeves from an old sweater and used them as leggings. Nobody, according to Danilova, wore leg warmers in the Diaghilev Company at that time; they weren't in existence. And thus leg warmers came into being. Other members of the company followed her lead, one by one. When the company went to London, the demand was such that Danilova ordered specially made pairs for herself and other dancers. The leggings, incidentally, were knit from oatmeal-colored yarn, a more suitable shade than that of the originally sacrificed sweater (a detail which Madame Danilova can't recollect).

Thus the inauspicious, if not apocryphal, appearance of leg warmers on the dance scene. It seems only fitting that their initial function was to warm the body specifically for the purpose of inducing weight loss through perspiration, rather than for other reasons. In fact, over the years the role of warmers has become increasingly obscure, which is quite in keeping with their debut.

One day, shortly before a class, I remarked offhandedly to an acquaintance that I was tired. It was a standard comment, meant to fill the sound void but not intended to be pursued further. I expected an equally perfunctory response, but the one I got was relatively thought-provoking: "I bet you wouldn't be so tired and would feel better in class if you wore more clothes. You know, it makes you sweat and feel all greased up."

Now I wasn't exactly underdressed, being fully equipped with a dance belt, leotard, tights, and ballet slippers. Conspicuously absent, however, were warmers. It just so happened that on that day I had decided not to wear them (it was a rather warm studio besides). Several thoughts struck me, but what really caught my ear was the word "grease," which Madame Danilova had used only the day before in a slightly different context. And in the various contexts of the word, I realized, rested the key to the true nature of leg warmers (a minor revolutionary linguistic breakthrough).

In one sense, warmers cause you to "get the grease out," the old "weight loss is fat loss" misconception that has already been dealt with here (I might add, parenthetically, that if fat *were* lost by perspiring, fat droplets rolling off dancers in class would make dance surfaces hazardously slippery). The other sense of the word "grease" is as a lubricant, something to oil and loosen up those rusting and creaking joints and tendons. This indirectly relates to the physiological benefits of heat, such as that produced by warming up. Muscle efficiency is enhanced at higher temperatures (in the nieghborhood of 102–103 degrees Fahrenheit), there is less resistance to stretch, and injuries are undoubtedly prevented by this muscular readiness.

Nonetheless, warmers are of limited and supplemental effectiveness even for warming. The best way to heat muscles is by working the muscles themselves. External methods of supplying heat—be they from a heat pad, heating balms, or a hot shower—provide warmth to a very superficial depth. The deep muscles used in turnout, for example, cannot be directly reached by these means (therapeutically, physicians employ diathermy, or deep heating methods). What warmers can do is insulate and retain some of the heat that results from muscular contraction. This is especially useful in cool studios, at the beginning of class when one's muscles are completely "cold," and in draughty backstage areas when there are periods of inactivity during a performance or rehearsal. As insulators, warmers are useful, provided they do not lead to overheating or dehydration. But they are never substitutes for a good preliminary warm-up or for reasonable dieting.

There are two other functions of warmers, widely accepted though less publicized. Whether one envisions oneself as too thin or too heavy, bulky warmers make excellent camouflage. How can an instructor see enough flesh to make corrections when her pupil is bundled up to the extent that she resembles a cross between an Eskimo and the Michelin Tire man? But the practice can be even more self-serving: it's the old "out of sight, out of mind" philosophy, supporting the specious syllogism 1) I can't see my overabundant thighs; 2) you can't see them either; 3) therefore, they do not exist. Even a dieter who is chronically rubberized may admit, under extreme duress, that though she knows the weight loss is not fat but water, she persists in wearing the suit as a "reducer" simply because "it makes me feel better," which is certainly a valid reason.

Finally, warmers are a fact of life in the dance subculture. Regardless of color or style (be they wool, acrylic, a blend, or rubber; store-bought, homemade, or improvised), warmers are a part of the way dancers are supposed to look. One might even question if it is possible to call oneself a dancer in their absence. And the more layered, the more eclectic, the more haphazard appearing, the better. Even a hot studio—with the sweat, the odor, the aching feet—can be a showcase for "high fashion," for what might be termed the "premeditated reckless abandon" look.

Consider the girl who suggested I cover up to grease up. As I recall her in my mind's eye, she is fully clothed for the workout. The underlying tights and leotard are not visible. There is a full-length navy acrylic warm-up suit, a rubber suit with the pant legs rolled up to mid-thigh and held with a piece of elastic, an additional pair of aqua warmers, and gym socks over those. Just in case there should be a sudden chill from the north, she has an aubergine sweater draped around her shoulders and wears a headscarf. And if by some chance she should sweat, she has had the foresight to bring along a small hand towel which she has draped fastidiously over the barre. So burdened with clothes is she that she could probably do an entire variation inside her self-styled shelter without there being the slightest indication of movement.

But what can I say? Admittedly, she is chic. And if one were to comment on her appearance, might she not say (like her equivalent walking late into a party wearing a designer turnout): "Oh, these old things? I just got up this morning and threw on

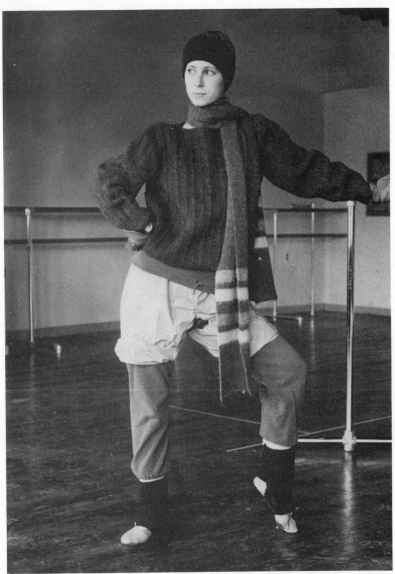

Figure 8: What did this warmth-conscious as well as fashion-conscious dancer
forget? A towel, draped fastidiously over the barre, just in case she should
happen to perspire.
(Photo by William H. Batson)

what happened to be there." Some people just know how to dress, I suppose (see figure 8).

So we owe a large debt indeed to Madame Danilova, who inadvertently inspired, for whatever reason, what has become a virtual necessity for dancers. Perhaps the import of that momentous invention can be rivaled only by the birth of the first dance bag. Is it even possible to imagine a world without dance bags, in which dancers would have to transport their lambswool and bandaids in attaché cases?

Foul Play with Food

THE LAXATIVE PURGE

Men live not on what they eat, but on what
they digest.

—Proverb

Historically, the use of cathartics or laxatives has been a mainstay of medical therapeutics. Purging (the elimination of waste from the colon), in fact, was one of the three basic treatments of ancient Greek medicine. The triad included bleeding (to get rid of the bad humors), starving (to prevent new ones from forming), and purging (to get rid of the rest, from whatever exit). This approach spread like wildfire over the Western world before it finally died out, and I mention it now only because some dancers still seem to subscribe to the latter two-thirds of the triad.

But let's skip back over the scummy waters of history even farther for a moment to analyze the roots of this practice. The ancient Egyptians believed that internal decay was a cause of disease; the obvious solution they reasoned, was to eliminate the source of possible decay in the intestines. Thus, the Egyptians became the all-time experts on enemas, and according to Herodotus: "For three consecutive days in every month they purge themselves, pursuing after health by means of emetics and drenches; for they think it is from the food they eat that all sicknesses come to men."[36]

As only historical luck would have it, the Egyptian soil was—and still is—a generous source of *Ricinus communis,* the castor oil plant.

Traveling from the Nile to the Thames, we find that an empty stomach and scoured intestines were also prerequisites in the athletic training of oarsmen in nineteenth-century England. The use of enemas and cathartics for a body "purification" was considered indispensable in bringing the organs of digestion to a healthy state of action. Getting into shape for those poor souls included vomiting and purging (antibilious pills, with salts,

59

senna, and camomile), forced sweating (mandatory Turkish baths and long daily runs clad in heavy clothing), and a ludicrous diet (almost raw beef or mutton, stale bread, no vegetables, and a minimum of liquid).

And how did this grisly discipline come to be regarded as the *sine qua non?* According to the medical commentator Sir Adolphe Abrahams:

> Because originally, feats and contests of pugilism, pedes-trianism, or oarsmanship were confined to professionals, men of the lowest class whose lives were given to sloth, gluttony, intemperance, self-indulgences of every kind and the violation of all laws of hygiene, and in them a drastic curtailment of their customary habits was the most salutary precaution that could be framed and enforced.
>
> When sporting contests became fashionable, the gentle-man-amateur passing from the rôle of patron to that of participant naturally adopted the methods of his profes-sional *confrère.*[37]

We must not forget that the athletes of yesteryear were a far cry from their present-day counterparts, whose fame is such that their endorsement is sought for everything from deodorants to foot powder. Even Galen, who took care of the Roman gladia-tors, held jocks in contempt. In his *Exhortation of the Study of the Arts,* he observed: "When athletes miss their goal, they are disgraced; when they attain it, they are not yet even above brutes."[38]

When the purification rite mutated into a dieting method is not clear-cut. Of twenty-four ballet scholarship students in two company schools in New York City, a third told me that they had used (or were using) laxatives for weight reduction or mainte-nance. Almost a fad with the younger ballet dancers, laxatives appear to be more commonly used in this age group than diuretics or self-induced vomiting; though for many who submit to self-abusive routines, the mode selected represents only a personal preference.

The inadvisability—not to mention the inconvenience—of

cathartic use may be overshadowed by the priority for maintaining a fat-free body. One fairly tall young dancer would take laxatives the day before her adagio class, since she felt self-conscious and guilty for being so large and wanted to give her male partners a break by weighing a bit less. Laxatives may be used to alleviate guilt or to atone for food indulgence or binging—as in the case of the young ballet corps member who steadfastly refuses to eat anything after seven in the evening and relies on laxatives if she is unable to uphold her resolve.

The foolishness may be carried to a degree of mind-boggling stupidity. One teenage dancer was overdosing herself on four tablespoons of Epsom salts per day before she discovered that fluid retention was completely offsetting the "positive" benefit of "getting rid of the food I had the night before." Another aspiring ballet dancer described how she took laxatives off and on "when desperate," particularly while reducing from 120 to 110 pounds (for a height of almost five feet four inches). Her regimen had entailed one laxative (Ex-Lax) before meals and two more pills after. She was taking as many as eighty pills per week when she finally stopped due to a friend's urging. It seems that the concerned friend (also a dancer) had an elderly aunt who had become "so messed up from laxatives that she had to wear a plastic bag." And as the reformed laxative abuser (who now just uses diuretics) reasoned: "You can't dance with something like that."

Even though the ancient Greeks did not have Ex-Lax, a wide variety of substances served them well (and not so well) as purgatives, such as large amounts of asses' milk and decoctions of melon, cabbage, and other plants, often mixed with honey. More drastic remedies were black hellebore, castor oil, and colocynth.[39] In general, cathartics act to increase the bulk and liquid contents of the feces by various mechanisms. Cascara and castor oil are irritants, producing rapid propulsion of the intestinal contents and thus preventing adequate time for the usual reabsorption of water. Inorganic salts (such as Epsom salts) and indigestible fiber act as so-called bulky laxatives, increasing the volume of the contents of the gut (the salts do this by drawing in water and distending the intestine, speeding up the transit time of the food). Mineral oil works essentially by lubricating, preventing some of the reabsorption of the fecal water contents as it passes through the bowel. Ex-Lax is a trade name of a laxative containing phenolphthalein, an agent widely found in proprietary nostrums. The precise mechanism of action of this cathartic remains to be determined (the cathartic effect of phenolphthalein was discovered in 1902 by a man named Vamossy, during a study undertaken for the Hungarian government to determine its safety as an additive for identification of artificial wines).[40]

Laxative abuse hampers the normal absorptive functions of the digestive system, increases the body's loss of potassium, and may lead to dehydration. Chronic overusers may ultimately develop atonic constipation, that is, a loss of adequate colonic muscular tone and a dependence on laxatives for excretory regulation. Cathartics have no place whatsoever in weight maintenance or reduction.

SELF-INDUCED VOMITING

Vomunt ut edant, edunt ut vomant.
(They vomit to eat, and eat to vomit.)
       —Seneca, *Ad Marcian,* xix, 2

The Romans are given the dubious honor of having invented the vomitorium, where the overzealous feaster could empty his stomach after a heavy banquet. Some, as Seneca described, combining epicureanism with gluttony, would return to the table after vomiting to reappease their hunger. The custom is no longer with us, but the emphasis on slimness for the female in our culture rivals that demanded of women in Epicurean Rome. Whether the practice was discretely transmitted through the generations or reinvented more recently, the vomitorium is still with us, though it may be only the toilet bowl in a campus sorority house.

When I first asked a group of ballet scholarship students

(between the ages of fifteen and twenty) at a large New York company school about vomiting as a means to maintain or lose weight, they cautiously exchanged looks until someone finally blurted: "You should have seen this place on Sunday nights [weigh-ins were on Monday]. Jeez . . ." She started giggling, and the previously uncomfortable silence erupted into agreement and slightly embarrassed laughter. The secret was out, confession was good for the soul.

Inquiring further, I learned that: "Nobody would eat anything past twelve noon, and the whole second-floor bathroom [of the women's residence] would smell so bad that you couldn't use it." Some would even make last-minute preparations, vomiting up Monday morning's breakfast before heading to the studio.

Everyone in the group overwhelmingly claimed to know "others" who commonly vomited (as well as used laxatives and diuretics). They were obviously hesitant to confess to those transgressions themselves, though a significant number of the young women present admitted to their participation by questionnaire and in individual interviews.

Aside from the natural repugnance that many people feel at the thought of forced vomiting, the possible deleterious effects outweigh even the aesthetic undesirability. Repeated vomiting (also called emesis) may lead to dehydration, body mineral and pH disturbances from the loss of acid stomach secretions, and even the traumatic tearing of the esophagus. This isn't to say that a large percentage of vomitors inevitably will be stricken with such maladies: contributing factors include the frequency of vomiting, the amount and type of retained dietary intake, and the activity and constitution of the person involved. And fortunately, Mother Nature generously allows us considerable leeway in our dietary indiscretions (see figure 9), as the stubborn persistence of our all too human species readily attests.

What is more bothersome than the possible detrimental physical effects, though, is the attitude that these dancers must have or develop toward their bodies, as well as the extrinsic pressures that contribute to making vomiting a viable alterna-

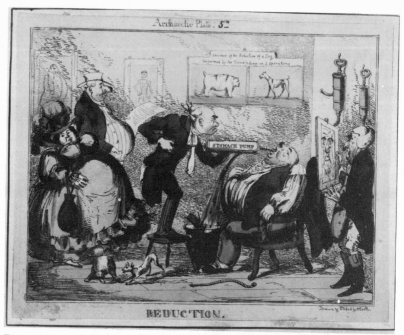

Figure 9: A nineteenth-century etching by H. Heath illustrates one of the many weight-reducing follies, the employment of a stomach pump. Two additional caricatures of the period depict the action of cathartics and emetics, antiquated mainstays of medical therapeutics that have been perverted even further for svelte's sake.

(Courtesy of the Logan Clendening History of Medicine Library, the University of Kansas Medical Center)

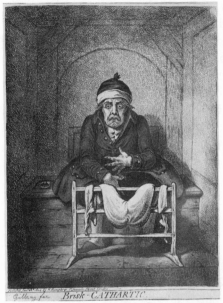

Brisk - CATHARTIC

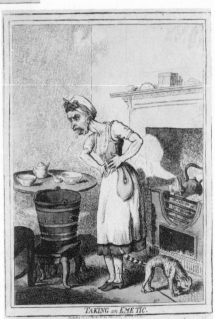

TAKING an EMETIC.

tive. Whether done only intermittently or adopted as a routine, vomiting may be taught and reinforced by the dance milieu. An eighteen-year-old ballet company apprentice detailed her concerted efforts to make herself throw up (an act which disgusted her and which she had always had difficulty doing, even when sick as a child). She combined various ingredients that dancer friends had told her would induce vomiting (including milk, mustard, salt, and pepper) only to find, to her dismay, that "it tasted good." Her experimentation with ipecac was also unsuccessful (due to her failure to drink ample amounts of water, necessary for the emetic to work). Thus, repeatedly thwarted, this particular dancer decided that vomiting wasn't worth the the effort, so she contented herself with using laxatives and diuretics.

A modern dancer in her mid-twenties who vomits three to four times per week recalls being "jealous as hell" over the vomiting of her best friend and roommate before embarking on the method herself, which she has now maintained for over seven years. Nonvomiters may feel quite resentful of their vomiting peers, though they might never be prompted to indulge in emesis themselves. One ballet student expressed personal conflict and irritation over her roommate's habit, though it was never openly discussed and the latter dancer made token efforts at being clandestine by locking the bathroom door and running both faucets full force during the process. The nonvomiter was concerned for her friend's well-being but also felt angry: "She's cheating—it's not fair," she told me.

An interview with another young ballet student brought out the same conflict. Aware of the practice while at a performing arts school, she did not force vomiting herself until moving to New York, where she faced more rigorous competition and professional demands. To make matters worse, instructors and peers considered the thinnest girl in her ballet class "gorgeous," though the girl allegedly "vomited all the time, pigged-out constantly, and couldn't diet." At that point the young dancer determined that there was "no reason I'm going to be heavier than everybody else."

During a six-month period, the seventeen-year-old vomited on a regular basis of at least three times a week, usually after the evening meal. She finally quit because of her growing disgust with it and with herself. Still, she was bitter at the injustice of it all—vomiting gave a competitive edge.

"It's cheating," she exclaimed, echoing her cohort's sentiments. "But they're just cheating themselves," she went on more quietly. The realization evidently not providing her much comfort, she became sullen.

"But you have to compete with them," I said.

"I just want to be thin," she said flatly.

This statement is coming from a female who is five-feet-five-inches in height and in agony over her weight of 102 pounds.

"You're thin now," I said.

"I don't think so, I feel heavy. It feels so much better when I'm 95. That's how I was this summer [the time of her vomiting regimen]."

"I don't think it's unreasonable for you to maintain your weight at 102," I said.

"I look horrible at 102."

Again I had rammed into the brick wall of self-perception and arbitrariness regarding the concept of beauty. Logic and reason would be of no use in arguing a point of health. The subjective question of beauty is nowhere to be found in medical texts.

Self-induced vomiting isn't something people are willing to talk about, as many participants feel embarrassment, shame, or even that they are "weak-willed." For others it may be a matter of course, a habit they are trapped in and almost compelled to maintain. In either event, it may be well concealed. An administrator of a ballet company school (students from this school had first informed me of routine vomiting prior to weigh-ins), when asked if scholarship students vomited to keep their weight down, replied: "Do I think it's done? I can't give you an answer because I don't live with these children and I am not aware of their habits when they leave here."

Another company school director told me: "I suppose it goes on, but we have not heard anything in particular, not at all. But I know they diet; I know some of them have weight problems and have diet charts and that sort of thing."

Still another administrator in a ballet school was somewhat more informed, but reluctant to come out with it, understandably wishing to avoid any implication of school or personal responsibility. It was a simple yes or no question: "Do your kids vomit?" but the answer wasn't quite that simple.

"Well, the school was weighing them in every Saturday, and then we found out that they were doing some special, uh, things of not weighing that much on that particular day, like not eating the day before or I believe someone said something about laxatives or something or other like that."

"But were they throwing up?"

"Not that I know of. I don't know."

"So what did you do?"

"Obviously they were doing something wrong, so we switched the day, the time of weighing, when they wouldn't know when it would be; so they wouldn't do anything that would be harmful to themselves—unnaturally."

Now that was a logical approach. Dance students do some things "unnaturally" in order to weigh less for a weigh-in; hence, if the exact time of the weigh-in is kept secret, then they won't know when to do their "unnatural" things and the problem will be solved. The rationalization was one which I did not wish to pursue further.

But let me not portray these teachers or administrators as ruthless Fagins, exploiting pathetic hordes of lost youths. Those who are aware of the situation (and truthfully, I believe that some are removed from the dancers to such an extent that they aren't) may be concerned and frustrated, and may even feel guilt about their implicit involvement. But the realities of the situation leave them impotent in effecting change. And there are practical concerns: the school must go on, potential and talent must be developed, the vacated spots in the companies must be filled from the ranks of the lower echelons. The weak will fall by the wayside, will be trampled under the advancing armies in pink satin shoes and chiffon skirts.

We must be careful neither to exaggerate the prevalence of self-induced vomiting among dancers nor to limit its presence to this population. Self-induced vomiting exists throughout all strata of our society. Whether it be the "flipping" of jockeys or the "dieting" of models, actresses, or housewives, this practice pervades, and is bred by, a culture that equates thinness with beauty and success.

I quote a female endocrinologist: "Take a female executive—your standard, terrific-looking, tough, put-together woman—and she goes to the bathroom and vomits after dinner. I don't think it happens to be normal to vomit after dinner. I'm not a big one for putting names on things—I just look and see if the behavior is healthy or not healthy for an individual. I think self-induced vomiting is not healthy."

With this statement I wholeheartedly concur. Self-induced vomiting is physiologically not a healthy practice. But there is a more important question that can't be answered as easily: Do psychologically "healthy" people vomit? Let us take a more personal glimpse of another vomiter before considering that question.

PORTRAIT OF A BINGER

Miss X is in her late twenties and is a modern dancer in a professional company. A dancer since childhood, she is a bright, articulate, college-educated woman, with a strong, well-proportioned, though slim, body of 110 pounds (for a height of approximately five feet four inches). One would be hard-pressed to compare her to some of her frail young counterparts aspiring to be ballerinas. She is older to begin with, and she is an established, seasoned performer. Although slender by most standards, she might be considered too heavy for classical ballet repertory in some companies, but for her type of dancing she requires the weight and the strength, and is aware that a weight loss of even five pounds is noticeably detrimental to her performing. She eats good food, has varied interests and talents, interacts well socially, and loves her work. She does not have any problems with cigarettes, alcohol, or drugs. Her problem is with food. Miss X is a bulimic, a food binger and chronic vomiter, who has been unable to get through a "clear" day (a day without vomiting at least once) in months.

Miss X describes herself as having been a "dieter" for as long as she can remember, consistently alternating between bouts of overeating and periods of semistarvation, agonizingly denying herself food when she knew she had to lose weight for professional reasons (she has never, however, weighed more than 120 pounds). In her mid-twenties she first learned a trick of the trade.

> I had eaten too much for dinner . . . and I was going through agony because I still had been trying to lose weight . . . and I must have been so stupid because I could never figure out why those two girls [sitting across from her at the dinner table and partaking liberally from the salad bar] stayed so tiny and ate three times as much as I did. So they told me. At first it was difficult—you have those hang-ups that you have to be sick, it's distasteful—but it comes up the same way it goes down, it's so easy . . . when I got to the point where I discovered how easy it was—that everything I put down I could put right back up again—it took a tremendous pressure off. There was no denying anymore.

A regime of chronic vomiting involves a certain amount of logistics, and bingers devise their own methods and food preferences. Miss X described different "grades" of vomiters: those who can eat a mouthful of food and throw it up, as opposed to those like herself who have to overeat considerably before emesis is possible. The vomiting can be induced by gagging with a finger down the throat or by developing simple muscular control. Miss X described her long torso and noted that food sits high in her stomach after a binge; hence, she simply has to push on her abdomen to initiate the expulsion of its contents. A dancer friend of hers has always had a more difficult time of it, and sometimes resorts to placing something distasteful on her fingers to cause herself to gag (usually a nail polish designed to discourage nail biting).

Binge foods are usually not exotic and often will consist of whatever is around the apartment. A very practical consideration is expense. Miss X makes a point of rarely binging on junk food, since "sugar binging gives you the shakes; it's a tremendous shock to your system." A cardinal rule is to drink lots of liquids on a binge, especially milk, says Miss X. And there are certain foods that one avoids; for example, one intent on regurgitation would be ill advised to eat a jar of peanut butter. I was informed that eating peanuts (with liquids) is preferable to eating peanut butter, but the latter can be managed in moderate amounts if it is consumed on warm toast. Following are exerpts from the interview, depicting her life style and relationship with food:

Vincent: Did you throw up today?

Miss X: Yes.

Vincent: After breakfast?

Miss X: No, after lunch. I almost consistently make it through breakfast [which had consisted that morning of a part of a cantaloupe, cottage cheese, coffee, and a variety of vitamins]. I usually binge at night after rehearsal.

Vincent: What did you have for lunch?

Miss X: Today I had a huge salad, then I had another salad, then I went out and got some chicken and some bread—I just ate about three good, normal meals—and then I had a box of fig newtons, over a quart of milk . . .

Vincent: Do you binge every day?

Miss X: I have been.

Vincent: What will you have for dinner?

Miss X: I don't know.

Vincent: Will you throw it up?

Miss X: I don't know; it's better not to plan those things.

Vincent: Do you eat when you're hungry?

Miss X: I have no idea anymore when I'm hungry and when I'm not.

Vincent: Do you enjoy eating?

Miss X: Yes.

Vincent: All that food?

Miss X: I enjoy it for a while, then it gets uncomfortable and it isn't fun anymore. When you get to that point, the whole world stops—everything is totally tuned out. My whole focus is food, that's it.

Vincent: What's the most you've vomited in one day?

Miss X: Six times. That's just about eating from morning until night.

Vincent: Don't you get tired?

Miss X: You get exhausted, but it just doesn't stop.

Miss X has watched her gradual progression from a once-a-week vomiter to her present state: "In the beginning stages my excuses were 'I have to keep my weight down for dancing.' But it's like a child that's grown into a monster; it's so much more than that now. I just can't blame it on my dancing—it's far bigger than that."

She tries very hard not to vomit on performance days, because "if I do a lot of heavy binging or throwing up, and if I take laxatives, I know that I'm shaky, and I can hardly see straight." If she can get through three or four "clear" days, she feels stronger, but that isn't enough reinforcement to break the vomiting routine; she's tried many times to maintain a diet without binging, unsuccessfully. Her addiction has reached the point where she has made excuses while out on a date so that she could go home and continue binging by herself.

Binging is by nature isolating—it takes time and is not feasible socially or in public places. But the binger is mentally as well as physically isolated. Few, if any, people may know the secret—not the family, not the choreographer, perhaps not even the spouse. In fact, one of Miss X's greatest fears is that someone will walk in on her during a binge. People are naturally shocked by such habits, and justifiably ill equipped to deal with a problem that can be quite a clinical challenge for a psychiatrist. For this reason, Miss X has been reluctant to reveal her practice even in close relationships with men. Only recently has she become open about her binging with close friends who are not bingers themselves.

Miss X knows other dancers who are bingers and describes them as all different, with different reasons for their eating disorder. She views her own problem as a disease of a hundred faces:

> One day it's because it's frustration, another day it's something else. And I'm wondering what it will take to stop; whether I'll be frightened to death at some point, because I ultimately know it's very harmful. . . . I don't think that the average person has to go out on a stage and be bigger than they are, and that's part of what's demanded of me. I'm constantly trying to transcend either my own emotions or my physicality—then I have to go home at night and face my physicality, my emotions—a lot of things I just can't handle. It's my way of tuning out, of not thinking, of blotting out absolutely everything.

And so she struggles with the frustration and the guilt ("five binges later, and you turn around and look at yourself, and it's really awful"). She doesn't want her binging to run her life—she sees the waste of energy involved in "putting two hours into something financially draining, mentally draining, physically draining." And yet, much as she would like to solve her problem: "The very fact of having to go back—which is the worst agony? Having to go back and be on a very restricted diet; I'm not looking to get rid of this problem and have another one to replace it."

Miss X says of herself: "I'm a good dancer, I'm strong, I'm reasonably healthy"—which makes her feel all the more terrible when young, admiring dance students ask her how she manages to keep so thin. "'Well, look at me—I eat thirty Hershey bars and ten dinners every night. That's how I keep so thin.' Is that what I'm supposed to say? So I don't answer them. I change the subject. I would never do that to somebody else."

THE DEFENSE

Miss X is a striking and extreme example, and by using her as an illustration I in no way wish to suggest that vomiting is necessarily addictive. This would be as ludicrous as claiming that all social drinkers inevitably become alcoholics. In our consideration of "normal" versus "abnormal" behavior, we might place her at one end of the following hypothetical continuum:

1) Anne came home for the holidays, and finding her mother's cooking so much better than college dormitory food, she ate too much at the family dinner. She went for a walk but with no relief. Finally, as a result of her stomach discomfort, she made herself vomit, something she had never done before.

2) Sue is dieting, and she has learned from a friend that she can vomit after a large meal if she loses her willpower and breaks her diet. She has felt guilty enough to do this about five or six times this year.

3) Gloria has always been a poor dieter, but has found that an effective way to lose weight is to vomit whenever she goes off her diet, which is often.

4) Miss X is a compulsive eater, binging on large amounts of food and vomiting afterwards. She doesn't know why she eats, but is unable to control her behavior, which at this point is detrimentally affecting her everyday life and relationships.

Since eating behavior depends on a variety of internal and external factors, at what point does one draw the line? Anne's behavior appears fairly understandable, but the question becomes one of degree. Anne overate one time and vomited, and Sue does it rarely; but then we get to Gloria and finally to Miss X, for whom the vomiting is extensive and is perceived even by her as a problem. The issue is complex, but we are being inaccurate in identifying the vomiting as the central issue. Whether or not vomiting is ever appropriate, it represents a response or a defense: perhaps a defense against heaviness, or against uncontrollable eating, or against failure in a job or competition. Vomiting isn't a disease, it's a symptom, and may equally result from an intestinal flu as from a distortion in body image.

Whatever the circumstances, with time a symptom such as vomiting may come to take on a life of its own. In a sense, all psychiatric symptoms are very much like an addiction, in that a whole new set of dynamics is set in motion by the presence of the symptom, and that the symptom itself may be sustained by factors quite independent of those which precipitated it to begin with. With vomiting, there may be an habituating effect. For example, a vomiter may feel constantly hungry and dehydrated, and because of that, will eat or drink more, thus bringing on the feeling of fullness, the guilt, and therefore the need to vomit again.

Margaret Mead insisted on the need to take into account the sociocultural framework of food habits, and this is easy to appreciate in the case of a model, a jockey, or a dancer. To a lesser extent, it applies to all of us, from the businessman who wants the physique of a professional athlete to the secretary who wants to look like a cover girl, all in the interest of greater happiness and success. A fifteen-year-old girl seeking a dance career may be entering a world in which the image conceived for women is a distortion of usual standards. If she lives in a dormitory where a significant number of her friends vomit before a weigh-in, one might not label her participation in that practice as "abnormal behavior." It is therefore much easier for me to conclude that her environment is unhealthy than to comment on the psyche of an adolescent girl.

Weight loss and maintenance can always be achieved through reasonable and conventional methods. However, if expectations are unrealistic, neither these nor hazardous and unconventional means will ultimately be of any use. I do not know of any dancers who, having attained their desired weight by vomiting, have then ceased the battle. They struggle constantly, reinforcing their own unhealthy patterns and behavior, victimized by their obsession. Whether vomiting represents normal or abnormal behavior is a subjective and perhaps academic question; that it is unhealthy is difficult to dispute.

Menstrual Themes And Variations

They don't menstruate . . . so what?
  —Lincoln Kirstein, in conversation

My first exposure to the extent of menstrual irregularities in dancers came about quite inadvertently. An eighteen-year-old student from a ballet company school asked me a general question concerning vitamins. After I mentioned that she might select a multiple vitamin with supplemental iron—since menstrual flow accounts for increased iron losses—the dancer concluded: "Then I suppose my friends and I can just buy the kind *without* the extra iron."

The absence of menstrual periods caused little concern and had not been evaluated by a physician, simply because the dancer did not consider her irregularity at all unusual. In the residence house in which she lived with other dance students, periodicity seemed almost a novelty. Continuing my inquiries into the menstrual patterns of young dancers, I encountered a surprising number of girls who responded to "Do you have periods?" with a naive shrug or the more pat—though somewhat obtuse—reply: "Yeah,—sometimes."

Agnes de Mille has observed that "certain great soloists have been lacking in even primary sexual functions and are known to have menstruated rarely in their lives."[41] From talking to past generations of dancers, it does appear that menstrual irregularities were common, though I suspect less so than they are today. A former principal ballerina recalled the extensive medical testing she underwent—including a visit to a clinic in Switzerland—for evaluation of menstrual dysfunction and apparent infertility.

"Nothing worked," she told me. "I didn't have my periods except when we were on vacation. If we weren't performing for a couple of months, maybe then I would have it once. Nothing worked until I stopped performing and went into teaching." (She is now the mother of three.)

We might go back even farther—quite a ways farther—to note

that Aetius of Amida (the first eminent Christian physician of antiquity, who made house calls in the sixth century) made the observation that dancers do not menstruate. He also noted this of emaciated women, barren women, and pregnant women, as well as of singers. In the case of the entertainers, either of song or dance, he reasoned that the menstrual blood was consumed by too much exercise (the singers in those days must have done veritable Las Vegas acts).[42] But conversely, many centuries before that, the reputable Hippocrates might have prescribed dancing as a cure for the failure to menstruate.[43]

Conflict and confusion about menstruation have abounded throughout the centuries; and naturally, man has made the most of his ignorance and dogmatism, with women bearing the brunt of the idiocies. Our medical predecessors were aware of the complexity and numerous contributing factors; consider the "shotgun" approach of the early nineteenth-century physician Marc Colombat de L'Isère, whose diagnostic checklist for failure to menstruate included: living in a low, humid locality; lack of sunlight; want of exercise; insufficient nourishment; fatigue; anger; disappointed love; celibacy; despair; jealousy; immoderate joy; "depressing passions"; "vivid emotions of the soul"; reception of bad news; a sudden fright; fear; sudden exposure to cold; the action of strong odors; ingestion of ices, sherbets, and cold drinks; and sitting on the grass, ground, or a stone bench.[44]

And if women dread visits to the gynecologist these days, a list of the elaborate and varied treatments of the past for failure to menstruate will leave them counting their blessings: fresh, dry air; nourishing food, particularly rich soups and roasts; wines and mineral waters (not bad so far); mineral water douches; foot baths; hip baths; warm enemas; aromatic fumigations; fomentations to the external genitalia; cuppings to the thigh; bleedings from the extremities; and leeches to the vulva.[45] Verily, the modern physician is part of a great tradition of menstrual bewilderment.

I have informally surveyed over a hundred aspiring ballet dancers in New York City by questionnaire. Of the fifty-five females in the group over sixteen years of age, only about a third described their menstrual cycles as regular; another third described them as irregular or intermittent; and the remaining 34 percent were not menstruating while actively dancing. Of this latter group, 14 percent had never had a period at all.

For a number of reasons this casual survey is not conclusive or even statistically significant: there was no control population for comparison; possible pathological causes of the abnormalities were not ruled out by medical evaluation; the use of a questionnaire instead of personal interviews always leaves room for ambiguity; and the population was small and certainly not random. I intentionally chose to investigate precisely the group in which I assumed problems of this nature would be frequent: young girls in highly competitive professional ballet company schools in New York City. Nonetheless, the results are striking, and they are consonant with data which is emerging about other female athletes as well as with what is regarded as common knowledge in the dance world anyway.

Because physicians experienced with dancers encounter menstrual difficulties so routinely, they are often more conservative in their approach to the dysfunction than others. Since the irregularity may often be viewed as part and parcel of dancing—with few or no ominous ramifications—the doctor may take a "wait and see" posture, with the only therapy a bit of needed reassurance. In comforting dancer patients, one New York physician explains that every profession has its own problems and that in the case of ballet, "the ovaries go to sleep."

Another physician uses a less tranquil and more movement-oriented trope for his dancers, telling them: "Your body's moving one way, and your ovaries are moving another way, and there's bound to be a clash somewhere along the line."

Simplistic explanations, but quaint, very quaint. Truthfully, I'm very supportive of the notion of personifying internal organs. Vividly can I visualize a yawning ovary, tucking itself into its pelvic omentum for a few winks, lulled by the soothing, rhythmic music of blood flowing through the inferior vena cava.

Or another, after being bounced around in an anatomical Waring blender (a lot of jumps in class), groping about to steady itself in a pulsating blur of dizziness, saying, "Phew, am I disoriented! Which way are the tubes?"

Certainly the metaphors serve their purpose, and resorting to them is unarguably easier than explaining the intricacies of the menstrual cycle, a task that many doctors face with as much reluctance as the patient who has to listen and feign comprehension. A New York fertility expert—a very skilled medical educator and writer—was attempting to explain the function of cervical mucus in response to a telephone question during a radio talk show. To simplify, he described the function of the secretions (which facilitate the transport of sperm to ovum) as "putting out a welcome mat." A reasonable effort, I thought, but the moderator interrupted him promptly with: "Well, I don't think we should get too technical for our radio audience."

Since that time, which was several months ago, I have pondered the question "How technical is a welcome mat?" And if a welcome mat is too technical, how on earth can one possibly talk about things like "follicular-stimulating hormone releasing factor" or the "hypothalamic-pituitary ovarian axis" to a group of dancers?

At any rate, before considering amenorrhea (failure to menstruate) or oligomenorrhea (few menstruations), one must first at least partially address the basics of normal menstrual function. One need not be an endocrinologist to understand the major highlights and interrelationships. And having given physiology a fighting chance, one becomes aware that the hormonal regulation of the female menstrual cycle is a fascinating and intricate piece of physiological choreography.

A LESSON IN FEMALE REPRODUCTIVE PHYSIOLOGY

For many females, the bleeding phase of the menstrual cycle may be the only indication that the cycle is occurring. To make it clear that various parts of the body are working overtime all along, let us use menstruation as a convenient starting point for a brief general survey, beginning with southernmost parts of the anatomy and working progressively north.

Menstrual blood represents a peeling off and shedding of part of the endometrium, the lining of the uterus. Throughout the cycle, the uterine lining proliferates rapidly, increasing in thickness and vessel networks, developing glands for the production of secretions. The growth and changes are in preparation for the possible fertilization of an ovum and the pregnancy which would ensue. Should pregnancy not occur, the beefed-up lining is sloughed, bleeding occurs, and the building up process commences from scratch.

The changes in the wall of the uterus are controlled by the hormones estrogen and progesterone, both of which are produced by the ovaries. Hormones are chemical substances which have specific effects on a certain organ or "target." In this instance, then, the uterus is the target organ, and its activities and changes are influenced by, and dependent upon, the ovarian hormones. Hormones, in effecting body changes, might be viewed as signals, instructing, modulating, and integrating the communications of one part of the body with another.

The major function of progesterone is to prepare the endometrium for implantation of a fertilized egg and for the maintenance of pregnancy, and its effects are for the most part confined to the uterus. In a sense, it antagonizes the growth effects of estrogen, or, rather, redirects the growth: estrogen stimulates the rapid growth of the endometrium, whereas progesterone stimulates the development of the uterine glands. In simple terms, estrogen affects the thickness of the lining, whereas progesterone affects the softness of the lining and its secretions, making the uterine wall conducive to implantation and support of the fertilized egg.

Estrogen, commonly regarded as the "female sex hormone," actually has a much broader job description. Aside from its effect on the uterine lining, it is responsible for many typical female characteristics. Breast growth and development, external female genitalia, the vaginal lining and secretions, and the deposition of body fat are all dependent on estrogen. The hormone also has a wide effect on general physiology, affecting blood proteins and fats and exerting influence on the vascular and skeletal systems.

Just as the uterus responds to the hormonal secretions of the ovaries, the ovaries themselves are subservient to the secretions of the pituitary gland (they are the target organ for pituitary hormones). The pituitary, about the size of a bean and located at the base of the skull, secretes multiple hormones which act on various targets for a variety of functions. For example: thyroid-stimulating hormone (TSH) stimulates the development and function of the thyroid gland; adrenocorticotropin (ACTH) does the same for portions of the adrenal gland (which itself is concerned with the synthesis and secretion of hormones called steroids); growth hormone (GH) is essential for tissue growth and repair; and prolactin is concerned with lactation in females. But presently we are concerned with the two powerful pituitary hormones that circulate in the bloodstream to affect the ovaries. Together referred to as gonadotropins, they include follicular-stimulating hormone (FSH) and luteinizing hormone (LH).

As its name implies, the function of FSH is to stimulate the growth of the ovarian follicle (the follicle includes the egg along with the cystlike structure of cells that surrounds it, serving to both nourish and protect the ovum as it matures). Luteinizing hormone is more responsible for the actual process of ovulation, in which the "ripe" follicle is expelled from the ovary into the Fallopian tube for possible fertilization by a sperm. The gonadotrophins, FSH and LH, do not produce all of their effects directly; rather some effects are determined by the type and relative amounts of the hormone secretion which they induce from the ovary (i.e., estrogen and progesterone).

Thus far we have traced the happenings in the uterus to the secretions of the ovary, which in turn result from secretions of the pituitary. The story does not end here, since the pituitary is controlled by a small section of the brain called the hypothalamus. The hypothalamus (involved with such crucial matters as water balance, satiety, and temperature regulation of the body) produces its own specialized hormones in nerve cells, so-called releasing factors, which regulate the production and secretion of pituitary hormones. There are separate releasing factors for growth hormone, adrenocorticotropin, thyroid-stimulating hormone, as well as FSH and LH. The releasing factors which control the gondaotropins have been called, originally enough, follicular-stimulating hormone releasing hormone (FSH-RH) and luteinizing hormone releasing hormone (LH-RH) (it has recently been suggested that a single releasing factor controls both FSH and LH).

The higher up we go, the more complicated things become and the longer the names get. The crucial point to be aware of, however, is that the hypothalamus is the bridge connecting the nervous system (the brain) with the endocrine system (the body secretions). Since the hypothalamus in turn receives input from the higher centers of the brain, which in themselves are modified and influenced by the outside world, any number of factors from the internal as well as the external environment may affect the normal sequence of events. Influences such as sensory stimulation, emotional states, drugs, and blood hormone levels all may alter the behavior of the hormone-secreting nerve cells of the hypothalamus, and hence the menstrual cycle.

The chain of command is more sophisticated than a strict superior-to-subordinate relationship. Unlike a one-way system, it is a circular one, integrated by a fine modulation of feedback, delicate hormonal signalings that may enhance or inhibit at various levels. For example, although the secretion of estrogen is the result of stimulation by FSH, high levels of estrogen shut off the production of FSH by the pituitary (negative feedback). Conversely, higher levels of estrogen actually stimulate greater production of the other gonadotropin, LH (positive feedback). Not only do the ovarian hormones affect the secretion of hormones higher up the ladder (via messages to the hypothalamus); the gonadotropins may also influence their own production, as high levels of FSH and LH act on the hypothalamus to suppress their own releasing factors.

Thus, the ovaries may communicate with the hypothalamus, with positive or negative instructions, as may the pituitary, and these communication lines are referred to as long and short feedback loops (it's helpful to think of distances here; the ovaries are much farther from the hypothalamus than the pituitary is). The sum total of all of these interrelationships is termed the hypothalamic-pituitary-ovarian axis (figure 10). Essentially, it's a system of checks and balances, insuring the integrity of the cycle. The alternative would be a bunch of glands haphazardly doing their own thing, an undesirable situation when something so basic as propagation of the species is at stake.

Figure 10: Simplified schematic summary of
Hypothalamic-Pituitary-Ovarian Axis

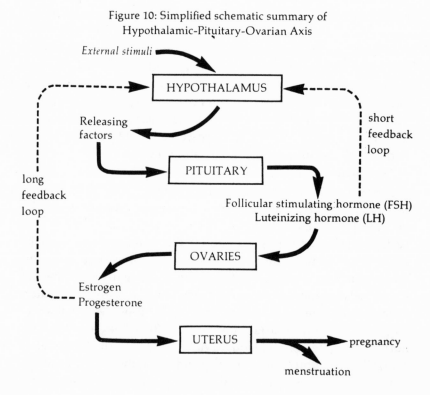

Given the remarkable control system regulating the menstrual cycle—dependent upon the synchronization and interrelationships of the hypothalamus, the pituitary, the ovaries, and the uterus—malfunctions may occur because of diseases involving the four principal players themselves or indirectly from other disease states. An overactive thyroid, for instance, may interfere with the development of the endometrium indirectly, since excess thyroid hormone promotes rapid elimination of estrogen by the body. Hepatitis, an inflammatory condition of the liver, may in some cases cause menstrual abnormalities via alterations in the normal metabolism of estrogen and progesterone.

MENARCHE, AMENORRHEA, AND IRREGULARITY

Obviously, problems with menstruation occur widely in the absence of "disease," and one need not be a dancer or an athlete to have firsthand experience. Let us examine several "case histories," using them as hypothetical models for nondisease factors that may be operating to produce menstrual dysfunction. The illustrations are factual, but I have substituted fictitious names.

> CASE 1: Sara is a nineteen-year-old scholarship student in a New York City ballet company school. She began dancing at the age of six, has been studying seriously since age twelve, and has not menstruated to date. She is five feet six inches in height and weighs 90 pounds.

Provided that there is no physical abnormality accounting for her initial failure to menstruate (primary amenorrhea), Sara might simply be called a "late-bloomer." Obviously she is well behind schedule, as the average age of menarche (the onset of menstruation) is roughly twelve-and-a-half years of age in the United States today. A hundred years ago, though, her case would have appeared less striking, as in those days menarche occurred most commonly at the age of fifteen or sixteen. From a study of 4,000 females in England in 1848, only 494 had begun to menstruate before the age of thirteen years and eight months; 632 did not begin until approximately their eighteenth birthday and beyond.[46] This trend toward earlier menarche over the past century (approximately three to four months earlier per decade in Europe) is associated with better nutrition and hence increased height and weight at correspondingly earlier ages.

It is well known that undernutrition delays the onset of menstruation; simple weight gain and increase in food intake have been shown to restore menstrual function in many of these instances after varying time intervals. But is Sara undernourished? Regardless of the beauty of her ballet line—whether one would consider her "slender," "skinny," or "too skinny"— Mother Nature has the final say-so regarding the timing of menarche. And according to the research of Dr. Rose Frisch and her coworkers over the past decade, it would appear that Sara—like other young dancers—is just too thin to start menstruating.

The hypothesis, which explains the effect of malnutrition on menarche as well as the trend for an earlier menarche, postulates a direct relationship between a critical "fatness" and the onset of menstruation. Through statistical investigations, it was found that at menarche, the mean weight of early and late maturing girls did not differ, although the girls who menstruated at a late age were significantly taller.[47] In other words, early maturers have more weight per height than their late-maturing counterparts. For the onset of menstruation, it was determined that a minimum of approximately 17 percent of the total body weight must be fat.[48]

Table 1 includes the ages, heights, and weights of twenty ballet student in New York City who have not yet undergone menarche. I have plotted these heights and weights on a chart (chart 1), devised by Drs. Frisch and McArthur and reprinted with permission, in which diagonal lines indicate approximate percentages of fat relative to total body weight (the lines represent percentiles of the ratio of total body water to body weight, an indicator of "relative fatness"). Seven of the girls (including Sara) are at or below the critical level of 17 percent body fat. All of the girls, however, are well below the 22 percent body fat marker, and it must be remembered that the figure of 17 percent represents a minimum for menarche. The average weight at menarche for American and most European girls is in the neighborhood of 102 pounds, which corresponds to a critical body composition of relative fatness in the range of 22 to 24 percent of weight.[49] The many different weights and heights of girls at menarche all represent approximately this range of percent body fat.

Thus, other factors aside, perhaps all of the girls have not yet menstruated because they just don't have a large enough composition of body fat. In the specific case of Sara, she would have to gain about nine pounds to attain the minimum 17 percent.

> CASE 2: Susan, a nineteen-year-old student of ballet, had her first menstrual period at age twelve, but has not menstruated at all for almost three years. Her weight at the time of her last period was in the neighborhood of 100 pounds. Currently she weighs 90 pounds and is five feet four inches in height.

Susan exemplifies a condition termed secondary amenorrhea, or cessation of menstruation after menarche has occurred (as opposed to primary amenorrhea, the failure of menses to appear initially, which should not be diagnosed before the female has reached the age of eighteen). Just as undernourishment delays the onset of menstruation, cessation of the menstrual period following chronic undernourishment or rapid weight loss has been well documented. Again, we may refer to the work of Dr. Frisch and her coworkers, who have demonstrated that established menstrual function ceases in older girls when fat levels fall below about 22 percent of body weight. For the female over sixteen who has already menstruated but has stopped because of low body weight, approximately 22 percent of the body weight as fat is indicated as the minimum for the restoration and maintenance of menstrual cycles.[50] From chart 2, another "relative fatness" graph, we see that Susan is well below the 22 percent minimum (in fact, she is even below the 17 percent body

Table 1

Age, height, and weight of twenty students of ballet in New York City who have never had a menstrual period

	Age	Height	Weight (pounds)
1)	12	5'1"	85
2)	13	5'4"	90
3)	13	5'½"	82
4)	13	5'	85
5)	14	5'2½"	96
6)	15	5'3½"	100
7)	15	5'1½"	90
8)	15	5'4½"	101
9)	15	5'4"	95
10)	15	5'2½"	95
11)	16	5'4"	98
12)	16	5'4½"	97
13)	17	5'2½"	95
14)	18	5'5"	95
15)	18*	5'6"	90
16)	18	5'3½"	97
17)	19	5'4½"	95
18)	19	5'2"	95
19)	20	5'5½"	102
20)	20	5'6½"	95

*Sara

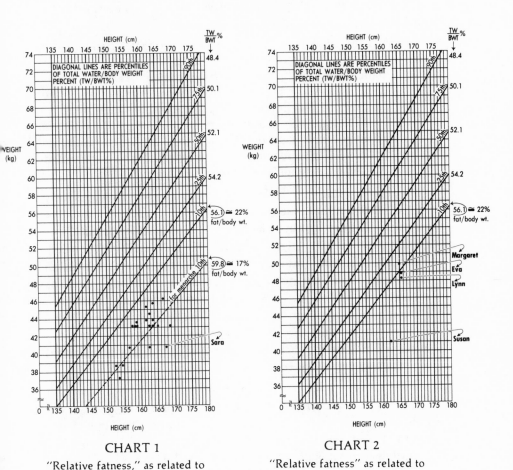

CHART 1

"Relative fatness," as related to menstrual onset.

CHART 2

"Relative fatness" as related to maintenance of normal menstruation.

fat minimum required for the initial onset of menstruation).

We might also apply the "relative fatness" argument in the cases of Lynn and Margaret:

> CASE 3: Lynn is an eighteen-year-old ballet dancer who had her first menstrual period at age thirteen, began dancing seriously at age fourteen-and-half, and currently menstruates about three or four times a year. She is five feet five inches in height and weighs 106 pounds.

> Case 4: Margaret is twenty years old, is five feet five inches in height, and has irregular periods. She weighs approximately 110 pounds and has observed that she hardly ever menstruates when she is below that weight.

Both of these females manifest menstrual irregularity which may be called oligomenorrhea, a reduction in the frequency of the menses (technically, this diagnosis is indicated if the intervals are longer than thirty-eight days but shorter than three months). When their heights and weights are plotted in chart 2, they both fall in the vicinity of the 22 percent body fat diagonal. Perhaps the fatness level is not adequate to maintain regular cycles, although there is irregular bleeding. That Margaret was herself aware of a "weight threshold" correlates very nicely with the observation that she is hovering at the borderline of minimal body fat necessary for regularity.

The above models seem reasonably straightforward, and it appears that "undernourishment" might contribute to a goodly number of menstrual difficulties encountered in the dance world, though the picture may in many instances be much more muddled. Darwin's observation that "hard living . . . retards the period at which animals conceive"[51] encompasses more than the obvious restraints imposed on fertility by poor nutrition. It is well accepted, and long a part of folklore and common observation, that interruption of the menstrual cycle may occur as the result of environmental stresses or changes. And here, one cannot rely on the statistical security of numbers and lines on a chart. The effect on a young woman's menstrual cycle of moving to New York City, or of competition in a company school, or of the pressures of a performing season can just not be plotted on a graph. Consider the not unusual situation illustrated by the following cases:

> CASE 5: Eva is a twenty-six-year-old ballet instructor in New York City who characteristically only menstruates during vacations from her dancing schedule. Her weight remains more or less constant at 107 pounds, for her height of five feet five inches.
>
> CASE 6: Kathy, an eighteen-year-old ballet scholarship student, had to curtail her dancing schedule for two months due to a back injury. During that time, she menstruated for the first time. Her weight of approximately 92 pounds (at a height of five feet two-and-half inches) has not varied appreciably over the past few months.

In both instances, abatement of dancing affected menstrual activity, resulting in resumption of periods in the former case and initiation of periods in the latter. When plotted on the "relative fatness" graph (chart 2), Eva is near the minimum postulated weight for maintenance of regular cycles, and Kathy is above the level considered necessary for initiation of bleeding, though below the minimum for maintenance (as a follow-up, Kathy has not yet had another period since resuming her classes). Nonetheless, the menstrual bleeding is not associated with variability in weight; rather, it appears to have a more direct relationship with dancing itself.

What is the nature of this dancing "stress"? Is it predominantly emotional—from the mental strains and pressures—or is it in some way related to changes in body metabolism, the increased work and sheer physical demands? What other factors are involved, and how may they relate to the critical percentage of total body fat? These are difficult questions and, at present, not completely answerable.

We might consider the somewhat analogous situation of other females athletes. Researchers have reported "irregularity" in distance runners, skiers, gymnasts, and other female athletes, as well as a significant incidence of amenorrhea during training.[52] It has been suggested that the incidence of menstrual irregularity increases with the degree of sustained physical exertion required. While this might be related to those intangible "stresses," it could as well be the consequence of a low percentage of total body fat, which is particularly characteristic of distance runners and gymnasts. We must keep in mind that the Frisch hypothesis is based on the relationship of body fat to lean body mass, not simply body weight. Thus, perhaps it could explain the amenorrhea in a heavy, muscular female swimmer. Although a far cry from a frail ballet student, and tipping the scales substantially, the swimmer might still have a relatively small percentage of body fat, which appears to be the significant factor.

Certainly the physical demands and emotional pressures of dancers are as great as or greater than those of other female athletes; and the professional necessity for a low percentage of body fat, particularly in the classical dancer, is much greater than in most other disciplines. Granted, the variables are multitudinous, the physiological system is complex, and individual variability is great. Still, we may comfortably accept at least one straightforward causal relationship: namely, "thinness"—in and of itself or along with the "stresses" of dancing—may be responsible both for the delay in the onset of menstruation and for the lack of maintenance of a regular menstrual cycle.

MENSTRUATION AND PERFORMANCE

The incidence of menstrual dysfunction among dancers is difficult to assess. The previous discussion, focusing primarily on a "susceptible" group, may not necessarily accurately depict the dance population in its entirety. Even among the aspiring ballet dancers surveyed, a third had completely regular periods. I suspect that a general survey of all dancers, including more mature ballet dancers, regional ballet dancers, and jazz and modern dancers, would reveal a lesser frequency of menstrual problems (though possibly still significantly greater than a control group of nondancing, nonathletic females). For the majority of dancers, then, the concern may not be menstruation per se, but dealing with symptoms that might accompany the cycle.

I have already alluded to physiological changes that occur as a result of hormone shifts. High levels of estrogen not only increase water retention, but also effect subtle changes in the permeability of small blood vessels, metabolism, and body temperature. It has been suggested that certain women might be more active because of peak estrogen levels. Some female athletes report that they perform best immediately after menstruation (during the postmense or estrogen phase), relatively well in the middle of the cycle (intermense or progesterone phase), and most poorly during menstruation, particularly the first two days. In one study, however, 46 percent reported no significant difference.[53]

Whatever the differences, the implication is that physical performance is not altered dramatically by hormonal nuances. Perhaps slight changes in efficiency may be discernible to a dancer keenly attuned to her physicality; water retention and cramping, however, are not easily overlooked.

Dysmenorrhea, or pain associated with menstruation, is a poorly understood condition, partially because of the subjective nature of the symptoms. Sports and strenuous activity can have both favorable and unfavorable effects on symptoms. It is generally assumed that females involved in regular exercise have fewer problems with menstrual pain and cramping, the exception being swimmers, in whom many investigators feel the prevalence of dysmenorrhea to be higher. In any event, the symptoms, if any, which arise, as well as the attitude and reaction toward these symptoms, will vary with the individual.

There is little evidence that training or performing during menstruation can unfavorably affect the cycle. Irregularity and dysmenorrhea do not necessarily have long-term harmful effects, and certainly neither class athletes nor dancers are going to avoid training or performing because of irregularity or discomfort. Full participation in dance should be allowed at all phases of the menstrual cycle; the final decision of whether or not to perform should always rest with the dancer.

Interestingly enough, dancers in Russia are guaranteed the option of three days off per month to accommodate menstrual symptoms, by order of the office of the minister of culture.[54] I learned in an interview with a Russian ballerina that—as in this country—most of the dancers are able to dance throughout the month. Nevertheless, a number of the Russian dancers, particularly the corps females, take advantage of the three-day allowance as a needed rest from their grueling schedule.

Perhaps this provision for calling in sick seems a luxury to corps members in this country. I find it hard to imagine a promising young dancer in a major company, working hard for soloist roles and facing stiff competition from her colleagues at the barre, approaching a choreographer with: "I think I'll skip class and the performance tonight. You know, it's that time of the month, and I feel a bit out of sorts."

At first glance, the three-day allowance in Russia seems a quite sympathetic and considerate gesture, but even the best of intentions may be perverted. A physician associated with the ballet world in Russia, who recently emigrated to the United States, told me a disheartening anecdote. A principal ballerina, known to have incapacitating menstrual symptomatology, did not see eye to eye with the artistic director of her company. By more than mere coincidence, her schedule worked out in such a way that her major performances nearly always coincided with the menstrual phase of her cycle. As a result, she missed performances due to "illness," a fact exploited by the director when appealing to the cultural ministry for her dismissal.

Dancers are disciplined and accustomed to dealing with professional adversity, be it bleeding feet, aching muscles, an injury, or menstrual symptoms. How can one who transcends emotions and physicality be brought down to earth by the monthlies? The general consensus is that the dancer who misses performances due to menstrual problems is definitely the exception. Often those who feel ill in the morning find they can "work through" their discomfort by taking class.

Of course, being a trooper doesn't make the problems disappear. If one were to talk exclusively with aspiring ballet dancers in New York and dancers burdened with a variety of menstrual complaints, one might conclude that there are two groups of dancers: those who have amenorrhea and those who don't but wish they did. I recall an interview with a principal dancer on one of her "rotten days." For her, the ramifications of the premenstrual period and days of bleeding were boundless. Aside from the depression, irritability, and cramping she experienced, her dancing technique was noticeably hampered. Fluid retention and swollen breasts threw her off balance during multiple pirouettes and required compensating adjustments. From the sound of it, she was a monthly walking disaster area.

"Have you ever missed a performance because of your period?" I asked (her career has extended over twenty years and is still going).

"Never," she said. She looked at me as if to say, "What a stupid question."

Developing as Dancers and Women: Peter Pan on Pointe

Very few dancers develop the bodies of
mature women; they keep lean in the
hips and flat-breasted, a phenomenon remarked on by all costume designers. It is
also a fact that the greatest performers,
the women best capable of communicat-
ing sensuous satisfaction, are in their
bodies the least sensual. In effect they
have sacrificed all organs of personal ful-
fillment and maintain and cherish only
the means for public satisfaction, the system of bones and sinews for levitation
and propulsion.

    —Agnes de Mille, *And Promenade Home*

I'm a dancer first, before anything else, so
I have to look like a dancer.

    —Member, New York City Ballet

Perhaps Agnes de Mille carried her generalization a bit too far,
but one doesn't have to be a costume designer to know that many
dancers, particularly those in classical ballet, keep lean in the
hips and flat-breasted. For the sake of argument, I shall state the
overwhelmingly obvious: dancers, particularly classical dancers,
must be slender. From an early age, aspiring ballerinas will not
be accepted into professional company schools if they are heavy
or appear to have that tendency. Similarly, heavy dancers will
not be accepted into ballet companies, and those who become
heavy will either shape up or ship out. Thus, the selection
process for "naturally thin" females in the world of dance.
Which explains why, after paying a pretty penny for orchestra
seats at Lincoln Center, City Center, or any other ballet house,
you do not often see women dancers with legs that look like
sausage rolls.

    That the selection is "artistic" rather than "natural" has been
established; regardless, selection in dance is a two-way street.
The dance may modify those selected in more than sociological

ways; in fact, it has the capacity not only of keeping one's physical development in a holding pattern, but also of causing one to regress physiologically.

This statement is not such a big jump from the relationships brought out in the previous chapter. We have seen that being "too thin" may delay the onset of menstruation or affect it once it has occurred. The onset of menstruation, though, is not an isolated phenomenon, as it reflects hormonal influences that may have other manifestations.

A LESSON IN "NATURAL" FEMALE DEVELOPMENT

Puberty refers to the transitional phase of development, the period of limbo bridging childhood and full maturity. The limbo is far from haphazard, and although the causes for the onset of puberty are enormously complicated and incompletely understood, there is a well-recognized order of progression.

Changes are heralded by enlargement of the nipples, occurring at about the ninth or tenth year. This is followed by budding of the breasts, enlargement of the external genitalia, the appearance of pubic hair, and the growth spurt. Hair under the armpits and changes in secretions of the vagina occur characteristically around the age of thirteen, with menstruation beginning within six months of these latter changes. Ordinarily, the adolescent growth spurt reaches its peak at about two months prior to menarche, then steadily declines and is virtually completed within one to three years after the first period.

During the adolescent growth spurt the greatest component of the weight gain is fat; body fat increases by about 125 percent, compared to an average 42 percent increase in lean body mass (muscle).[55] The priming of the ovaries for reproductive function is somehow triggered in relationship to this change in body fat composition. Well before menarche, hypothalamic releasing factors begin to stimulate the secretion of FSH and LH by the pituitary. Consequently, estrogen production begins, and the levels increase until sufficient estrogen is present for menstruation to occur. Usually at the beginning, however, no ova are produced, because for perhaps a year or two there is not enough LH to induce ovulation and allow complete reproductive potential.

As estrogen in increasing amounts will affect the lining of the uterus, so will it influence the development of the breasts. Prior to puberty, breast growth proceeds at the same rate as the growth of the rest of the body. During puberty, under the influence of greater quantities of circulating estrogen, the ductal system and the supporting fatty tissue of the breasts grow faster than the body in general. Although breast buds and pubic hair may appear two to three years prior to the first period, actual enlargement of the breasts and growth of the pelvis (including the accumulation of fat on the hips that contributes to the normal female contour) do not begin to occur until approximately one year after menarche.

THE PUBERTY HOLDING PATTERN

Sara and the other dancers who are "late-bloomers" will be lean-hipped and flat-breasted, and not necessarily because these are family traits. Though chronologically they may be eighteen, nineteen, or even in their twenties, they preserve the body configuration of an adolescent who has not completed the transition through puberty. They simply don't have enough estrogen or other hormones to kick things off, so, like Peter Pan, they can get older without really growing up.

Late maturers, with longer legs and narrow hips and less relative fatness, may be better suited than others for a variety of athletic disciplines, and the success of females with these characteristics might well contribute to the higher average age of menarche which has been reported in female athletes (of national and international caliber).[56] Regardless of other criteria, late maturers have a competitive advantage with respect to selection by professional company schools. This point is well illustrated by the words of a professional ballet school administrator with over four decades of experience in auditioning young girls for a potential career in ballet: "Our teachers . . . have a feel for a little girl's body that is already really a little bit too plump for the age. It's very subtle, but it's there. . . . There are some girls that are really developing very fast at a very early age, and we worry that that development is going to continue. And you can see that the girl is going to be a big—you know—well-developed, well-endowed girl."

So, if talent is a plus factor, along with flexibility and technique, estrogen isn't. The success of the selection process may not represent a self-fulfilling prophecy so much as a self-inducing one. Accept someone who is a late maturer to begin with, immerse her in the weight-obsessive culture, and you can be fairly sure of delaying her development still further. Thus, the "feel" has little to do with an ability to identify "naturally" thin girls. The need to start classical dance training at a young age involves more, it seems, than the development of technique.

If it is advantageous for a female ballet student to mature sexually later than the general female population, this isn't the case with males. During the years of active growth, male athletes are usually ahead maturationally compared to their nonathletic peers, and generally the good performers are more advanced than the poor performers.[57] Selection criteria and the demands of dance for the male will not as likely run a collision course with hormones.

PAST PUBERTY AND SHIFTING INTO REVERSE

Even long after the onset of menstruation and progression through puberty, women may revert back to abnormal or more immature hormone levels and patterns as a result of significant weight loss. In severely emaciated women with anorexia nervosa, a variety of hormonal changes occur, with a wide range of consequences (many, or perhaps all, of these changes may be due to nutritional deprivation). Women who have lost enough weight to cause menstruation to cease have been found to experience similar, though less severe or extensive, changes. Low body weight in females may correlate with abnormalities in the regulation of body temperature, changes in water conservation, and variations in hormone levels as well as in organ responsiveness to hormonal signals. Simple weight loss per se is enough to result in dysfunction of the hypothalamus, thus affecting secretion of gonadotropins by the pituitary and ultimately affecting levels of estrogen and other hormones.[58] Whatever the specific mechanisms involved, the changes are definitely related to the fat content of the body, and at least some of the dysfunction involves changes at the level of the hypothalamus or higher. "Related" covers a lot of ground and ignorance, and there are obviously message systems and communication lines in the body which persist in eluding investigators.

Clearly nutrition is of prime importance in hormonal regulation; the human female needs adequate energy stores to meet the increased demands of pregnancy and lactation. Researchers investigating the San tribes in Africa have demonstrated a seasonal variation in fertility according to variations in nutritional status among this hunting and gathering population.[59] And although it is commonly believed that malnourished populations have high fertility rates, this is not the case (the issue is often clouded by the absence of contraceptive practices in underdeveloped nations). In India, for instance, the mean interval between pregnancies in poor income groups—in which contraceptive practices are not employed—is thirty-two months. The causes include delayed puberty (diminishing the years of reproductive ability), decreased potential fertility (amenorrhea without ovulation), a greater number of miscarriages, and a higher percentage of mother mortality and stillbirths.[60] Mother Nature just may not view an ethereal ballerina as a good reproductive risk. On stage she may transcend artistically; physiologically, it's another ballet altogether.

THE METAMORPHOSIS CONSIDERED

For their part, most eighteen-year-old ballet dancers are not very concerned with their reproductive capabilities, and as far as breasts and periods go, many young dancers don't feel exactly heartbroken about the absence of either. Mature dancers are more likely to prefer more breast tissue with age, as the dichotomy between the dancer's and the woman's body becomes more pronounced and professional priorities begin to shift. But, as I have shown, a number of young dancers view maturation and physical development as a definite career threat (this paranoia may be justifiable), and some face the approach of menarche and breast growth with considerable dread and apprehension. Adolescence implies much more than hormone changes, and physiological developments must always be considered in light of the individual's socialization and, hence, perceptions and attitudes toward self. The dance world may shape the mental development of the dancer just as much as it does the physical.

Consider Jane, a twenty-six-year-old dancer in New York City, who began studying ballet seriously as a child but prefers working in jazz. At five feet four inches, and weighing 109 pounds, Jane doesn't see her body as that of the "ideal" ballerina. Following are excerpts from an interview:

Vincent: How do you feel about your body now?
Jane: I'm glad that I'm a jazz dancer and not a ballet dancer.
Vincent: Why?
Jane: Because as thin as I get, I have sort of—I don't know—a sexy body. And ballet dancers don't.
Vincent: So you want a sexy body.
Jane: I can't help it, what can I do? [Laughter] How much weight can I lose? [More laughter] You know what I'm saying.
Vincent: (politely) You're . . . uh . . .
Jane: Yeah, no matter how thin I get—I mean my arms will become pins, and I'll still—my bones will stick out to nothing, and I'll still have, uh . . .
Vincent: Go ahead. Say it.
Jane: I'll still have, you know . . .

[In this roundabout way, we finally established the obvious fact that Jane has a substantial bustline and a curvaceous body contour despite her thinness. We next discussed her initiation into the ballet world.]

Jane: I had always been an extremely thin child. I was incredibly thin. My mother was afraid for me, and I was at ——— [company school] and everything was great there, and then I started getting pressures and I left.

Vincent: What kind of pressures?

Jane: Well, I was on scholarship. I was only nine years old. And I hated it.

Vincent: Were you thin then?

Jane: Terribly.

Vincent: Because of the pressures?

Jane: No, I was just a very thin girl.

Vincent: Then you wouldn't feel pressure about losing weight if you were naturally thin.

Jane: No, but I always remember being told "Stay this way. Never gain weight, because you'll never have any troubles."

Vincent: Except you were growing [the growth spurt comes at this age].

Jane: But I was growing, and they were telling me not to eat, not to do this, so I left, and stopped dancing for about four years, and then I gained a lot of weight. [Then] I got my period—I was very young, about twelve or thirteen.

Vincent: How did you react to your first period?

Jane: I was relieved. Because I remembered thinking, "Now I'm going to get breasts."

Vincent: So you wanted breasts?

Jane: Oh, yes.

Vincent: That isn't the usual . . .

Jane: Because I wasn't dancing, remember? I stopped dancing [between the ages of nine and fourteen].

Vincent: So you think if you had continued dancing you wouldn't have wanted breasts?

Jane: Well, maybe. Because I would have been around girls who weren't developing. I was around girls who *were* developing [in public school]. But the most incredible thing is that I developed very quickly. I went from a skinny little girl to this .

From looking at pictures of herself as a child, Jane thinks she might have had a very good ballet body, because she was "thin and long." And, she believes, had she not taken the hiatus from classical dance, she might have adopted "a ballet life style." Had she remained in the company school, maintaining her "natural thinness," would her bustline be the same as it is today? Conceivably her puberty (and onset of menstruation) could have been delayed, in which case she wouldn't have developed that bustline as soon as she did. But can a woman genetically destined to have large breasts actually develop a different body configuration because of involvement in dance? The question boils down to whether or not the alterations in developmental progress are temporary or permanent.

This isn't the kind of question that is easy to study, so we can only make educated guesses based on empirical observations. The general consensus among endocrinologists and gynecologists is that it is "never too late" to develop breast tissue, provided there are the appropriate hormonal influences. One gynecologist cited the example of a patient who had an undiagnosed congenital abnormality and, consequently, extremely low estrogen levels. After the diagnosis was made and estrogen replacement administered, the woman began her breast development, at the age of fifty-six.[61]

Another gynecologist and researcher related her experience in following several dancers with delayed puberty, some of whom didn't begin menstruating until their late teens and twenties. After gaining adequate weight, she said, they seem to go through a "second puberty." "They suddenly start to develop. Their breasts start to develop, they put on weight, and they look absolutely normal. They go through a metamorphosis—it's amazing."

Of course, ultimately we are dealing with a question of more import than breast size or hip contours, that of reproductive capability.

In the last chapter I cited the example of a principal ballerina plagued throughout her career with menstrual dysfunction and infertility, which disappeared when she retired. It has been observed that in extreme cases of anorexia nervosa, reproductive potential and normal menstruation occasionally do not return despite weight gain, for reasons not known. But again, it seems that as far as the dancer is concerned, the halt in reproductive capability is just a stall. As the gynecological researcher stated: "I think ballet dancers have a prolongation of their prepubertal state, and that puberty is just delayed; or they revert to a prepubertal state if they've already started menstruating. And I think that most likely it will turn out to be a reversible thing that will have no long-term effects. That's my impression. I don't know."

The prevalence of hormonal modifications in female dancers is impossible to ascertain, and possibly it is of only academic interest. For the dancer, the most significant aspect of hormonal patterns is likely to be their relationship to weight control. A nineteen-year-old dancer with delayed puberty will wage a different war with food than her more curvaceous counterpart, who has undergone menarche and developed more "female" contours. And the mature dancer, who is no longer in a hormonal holding pattern, may find weight control a much more difficult task than she did when she was training in professional school. With a change in hormones, realistic body expectations may be transformed into unrealistic ones.

Consider the case of Ellen, an eighteen-year-old ballet scholarship student who has fairly regular menstrual function. According to a teacher, Ellen has "trouble with her weight." Currently weighing in at 115 pounds, she thinks she looks and feels good at 107, but the consensus is that she must get down to 100 pounds, especially if she wants to be accepted into the company (she is almost five feet four inches).

Ellen has been in New York for less than three years and underwent most of her sexual development while dancing regionally. Her goal is to look like a good friend in the school, a young woman "who looks like a fifteen-year-old" despite the fact that she is older than Ellen. The friend began ballet training at an early age at an East Coast performing arts academy, and although she is an inch taller than Ellen, she has no problem attaining a weight of 100 pounds (she would like to stay around 92, however).

"I would give anything to look like her," Ellen told me, and I believe her. Ellen has virtually tortured herself with laxatives, vomiting, and semistarvation. At the time of our interview, she was pursuing a ridiculous dietary regimen composed predominantly of liquids and diuretics.

In the meantime, Ellen's friend expects her first period one of these days, though she isn't exactly holding her breath.

Two to Tango: Partnering and Sexuality

Dancing represents sex in its least costly
form, free from imprisonment and free to
a great extent from the emotional responsibility and, above all, as a sure thing,
independent of someone else's pleasure.
In other words, it means freedom from
sex. The forces which impelled women to
the austerity of the church operate to
form the great dancer. In a strange trans-
mutation dancing is a form of asceti-
cism—almost a form of celibacy.
   —Agnes de Mille, *And Promenade Home*

My experience with these girls is that
they couldn't care less about sex. Even
the ones that are married, I think, have
very little sex life.
   —Physician, New York City

A common misconception equates physicality with sexuality.
The dance is not necessarily sexual, nor do dancers have to be
sexual beings. The absence of sex is perhaps best appreciated in
abstract, formalistic pieces, where male and female are inter-
changeable as androgynous forms in space. But even when
traditional romantic motifs dominate, a classical dancer need not
cast alluring glances at the men in the boxes—a tactic Fanny
Cerrito occasionally resorted to—to evoke sensuality. As André
Levinson has pointed out, the sexuality is in the movement itself:
". . . what one might also term the classic dancer, is purely
functional, serving to facilitate the mechanism of her art. Hence
its non-sexual appeal."[62]

Many may find it difficult to separate the work of the artist
from the life; the inclination not to do so may be quite
overwhelming—such is the power of the magic. The manufacturer's representative in the fifth row—entranced by the pas de
deux from *The Sleeping Beauty*—might squeeze the hand of the
spouse of twenty-five years sitting at his side. Afterward, in the
glow of the streetlights on Broadway, struck by the intensity of

the blueness and the time-worn but persistent sparkle of her eyes, he might be prompted to say things not said since the days when he was cocaptain of the football team and she played saxophone in the marching band at Paseo High School. Aside from an evening of watching fine dancing, these little luxuries alone would be worth the admission price.

But frankly it isn't really fair to expect as much from the Prince and Aurora once they've taken off their makeup. The Prince's real heartthrob may be waiting at home, or might be that loathsome wicked fairy. And though the two dancers hold one another so lovingly, perhaps their sexual preferences don't even jibe; they may feel ambivalent—or even hate each other's guts. Aurora may emerge from the stage door more drained than a boxer finishing a gymnasium workout. She may walk home alone, past the unrecognizing eyes of the manufacturer's rep and his wife, facing the prospects of no other company besides a Jacuzzi, a flannel nightgown, and a hungry cat to feed.

In sexual attitudes and behavior, the physiological and the psychological are welded into a human alloy. Because of the subjective nature of sexuality, I initially found myself hesitant to discuss it here, but not only because of the lack of meaningful or pertinent investigations or statistics. What made things worse was the creeping, paranoid suspicion that at this spot (the shortest chapter in the book) the reader would begin to pay more attention. I could already visualize a prospective buyer standing in a bookstore, thumbing through immediately to this section. Which undoubtedly accounts for the fact that my writing of this segment has been accompanied by the almost continual sensation that an insect of some sort is crawling under my collar.

Regardless, the topic is worthy of some mention, as I have been struck by how often the notion of asexuality has surfaced in conversations and interviews. Female dancers are not necessarily very sexually oriented. Certainly I would not be so foolhardy as to generalize concerning sexual patterns and attitudes of all dancers; the opening quotations must be taken for what they are—subjective impressions from one dancer and one physician.

Wishing at all costs to avoid deep-seated psychological explanations for these impressions, I want nonetheless to consider some aspects of the dance subculture that might directly or indirectly influence the sexual behavior of dancers. How a particular dancer might react to or be influenced by these factors is an individual concern, defying generalization.

SUBLIME SUBLIMATION

Socialization aside, the sheer physical work of dance might serve to dampen sexual preoccupations. Whether the diversion of sexual instincts through dance represents an unconscious choice or whether it is simply an incidental byproduct of the profession is of no matter. Regardless of his motives or psyche, I doubt that Casanova would have had much to brag about had he spent his afternoons training for the Boston Marathon. A professional ballet dancer might have eight performances a week for weeks on end, a demand which does not lend itself to carousing until the wee hours of the morning. As a young dancer told me: "Most dancers, when they come home from a day's rehearsal, just don't have the energy to go out and be social butterflies."

For a well-respected jazz teacher and performer in New York, the physical energy expended in dance is very definitely related to sexual energy. Having trained and performed as a classical dancer, she considered the situation of the aspiring ballerina: "I think they don't realize yet that the energy is sexual energy, and that it can become sublimated if you stay in the ballet, or be conditioned other ways... I didn't have sexual thoughts as young as most people, because my whole world was the ballet, and you see, without realizing it, that kind of physical exercise was releasing the tension anyway, so I wasn't aware of it. I wasn't aware of the tension because it was being released."

She notices pronounced variations in her own sexual cravings as related to her dancing schedule: "I know that as long as I dance every day, I'm on a very even keel sexually. But if I stop dancing for two weeks, all I want to do is have sex. I'm so aware, my energy is so intense, God help my husband . . ."

THE SEXUAL COCOON OF THE SOCIAL CATERPILLAR

Many young dancers, despite their interest in the opposite sex, find that the dance cloister has put them in a bit of a quandary. Even if they have the time, the type of social life they desire is simply not readily accessible. The well-insulated dance community may become a cage. Add to this the poor ratio for socialization (the preponderance of females to males), as well as a certain percentage of homosexuality, and things can become tougher.

Said a company apprentice: "Gay men can make things kind of difficult. The dance world is a pretty tight world, and you see so many of these people every day that are connected . . . and you don't have that much time to get outside social contacts."

Quipped another about her social life: "We don't know what to do about it sometimes. What are we supposed to do, stand on a corner? We joke about it a lot."

PROFESSIONAL PRESSURES AND PRIORITIES

Avoidance of social involvement may for some be rationalized as a means of guarding against a potential career threat. One young scholarship student told me she stopped seeing her boyfriend because he demanded too much of her time; not himself a part of the dance world, he didn't, she claimed, "understand" her priorities. A ballet company member in New York City summed up these feelings as follows: "[Some dancers] feel that getting involved would take away time from their dancing, in which case they wouldn't work as hard, they wouldn't get as many parts, they'd start losing their technique. And in the company it was—not so much now—but it was taboo to get married or even have a boyfriend."

Sounds a bit like shades of *The Red Shoes.* Marriage to both dance and a man may very well be viewed as mutually exclusive, either by the dancer or by her artistic director. The conflict between family and career is not by any means unique to contemporary women in dance, but for the dancer the problems are somewhat special. A professional ballerina who took a hiatus in midcareer to have a baby commented on the company director's reaction: "He would have preferred that I wasn't pregnant. Probably he would have hoped that it would have never come into my mind. Artistically he's right; I mean, what can he do with a pregnant sea nymph?"

Indeed, a pregnant sea nymph is the choreographer's problem, but ultimately the decision to have a child rests with husband and wife, and may entail considerable professional sacrifice. Consequently, most professional dancers will place family thoughts on the back burner, at least while they're in their twenties.

BALLETIC PASSAGES

Many of the young girls in New York City who are seriously pursuing a career in ballet either graduated from high school early (compressing four years into three), attended a professional performing arts school, or left their high school studies incomplete (often to be finished by correspondence or equivalency examinations), thus bypassing typical high school socialization. Not unusually, they dated either very rarely or not at all in high school; some were just "not interested," others "too busy," even though they wanted to go out and were often asked.

From talking with large numbers of these students, patterns of maturity emerge as almost characteristic of the subculture. When young, the dancers may be more precocious than their peers. Many dance in regional companies, interrelating socially with older dancers either as performers or in dance class (if talented and technically advanced for their age, they rank as the youngest members of their classes). High school activities may seem to them juvenile and a waste of time, a perspective illustrated quite well by Agnes de Mille: "I was fourteen, and I had found my life's work. I felt superior to other adolescents as I stood beside the adults serene and strong, reassured by my vision."[63]

With advancing age, however, the effects of the cloister

become more manifest. In high school the precocious dancer is less involved with her nondancing peers, anxious to leave school behind and get down to the business of dancing. At eighteen, nineteen, and twenty, many seem to lag a bit behind their nondancing counterparts, who, having socialized more extensively in high school, have now gone on to more broadening experiences at colleges and universities or the working world outside of the dance.

The priorities often seem to change in their thirties, when some ballet dancers find that the restrictiveness of their life style has led them deep into a blind passage. Dancers are neither more nor less vulnerable to career or life crises than anyone else, with one unfortunate exception: at the point when the career of a female professional may be just starting to blossom, the ballet dancer is rapidly becoming deadwood. Once again, I quote Agnes de Mille:

> Whatever the rewards the dancer knows in place of the usual emotional and sexual associations, she is frequently assailed by doubts in her late twenties or early thirties. Even the very great know these morbid spells. The needs of the heart cannot be cheated forever. The dancer grows frightened. The dancer realizes suddenly she is a spinster and aging, no matter how fast she gets around the room. The life of merciless effort, the dimming chances of permanent fame, exhaustion and the growing comprehension of what old age means to a fading athlete without family or home suddenly terrify even the staunchest. The conviction grows that the sacrifice has been too much and perhaps not necessary. There is many a volte-face at this point and a marriage with at least one child in a frantic effort to put life back on balance.[64]

DELAYED PUBERTY AND SEXUAL SPECULATIONS

The loss of normal sexual desires is a prominent and well-recognized characteristic in the severe emaciation of anorexia nervosa. Does the low amount of "sex fat" in some dancers influence sexuality from a hormonal basis?

Again take the hypothetical case of the nineteen-year-old dance student with delayed puberty or the young woman who has reverted to an immature hormonal pattern in association with low body fat. Remember that, aside from influencing menarche and breast growth, estrogen also affects the type of cells lining the vagina, as well as the type of secretions. Without appropriate stimulation from estrogen, sexual relations could be uncomfortable, or less comfortable—a physiological fact that might indeed discourage sexual activity.

In dealing with something as subjective as sexual drive, it is quite difficult to disentangle physiological and psychological factors. We have seen, though, that low body weight may affect the levels of hormones in the body, and we can assume that, in light of the relationship of hormones to sexual development, their altered presence may be manifested in the scheme of things. That the effect of such changes may be behavioral as well as physical is certainly plausible, though speculative.

Anorexia Nervosa and the Anorexoid Dancer

In the month of July she fell into a total
suppression of her Monthly Courses
from a multitude of Cares and Passions
of her Mind . . . From which time her
Appetite began to abate, and her Digestion to·be bad; her flesh also began to be
flaccid and loose, and her looks pale. . . . I
do not remember that I did ever in all my
practice see one, that was conversant
with the Living so much wasted with the
greatest degree of Consumption (like a
Skeleton only clad with Skin) yet there
was no Fever, but on the contrary a cold-
ness of her whole Body.
—Description of Mr. Duke's daughter in
St. Mary Axe, who became ill in July,
1684, in her eighteenth year, from *Phthisiologia: or, a Treatise of Consumptions*, by
Richard Morton, 1689

In a game called The Ballet Company, the object is to attain the status of prima ballerina assoluta by moving a playing piece around a board blanketed with a variety of professional obstacles (see figure 11). If one happens to roll a six on the first toss of the dice, landing on a square which orders the procurement of a Refrigerator Card, one might pick up a card saying: "Avoid eating for two entire weeks. Company sends you to a psychiatrist who diagnoses anorexia nervosa. Lose 1 fame card.[65]

Thus, as Richard Morton is commonly credited with the first description of anorexia nervosa (1689) in the medical literature (see figure 12), to my knowledge the first published reference to anorexia nervosa in context of the dance is on the aforementioned Refrigerator Card, published in 1973. That some dancers carry their weight obsession "a little too far" is well recognized in dance circles; and although most teachers and choreographers feel that the majority of weight problems are on the heavy end of the spectrum, the "too thin" dancer is highly visible.

The questions then arise: Is anorexia nervosa—a syndrome

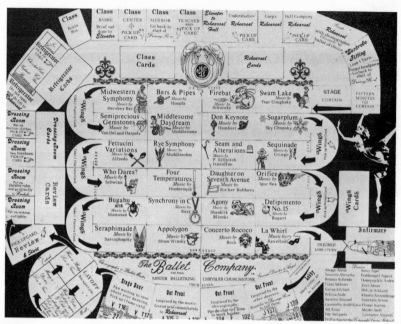

Figure 11: Reproduction of the game board of The Ballet Company Game, which contained (in a Refrigerator Card) the first published reference to anorexia nervosa in the context of the ballet world.
(Courtesy of Stetson Enterprises, 155 West 68th Street, NYC 10023)

characterized by self-induced starvation leading to profound weight loss—more prevalent in the dance world than in the general population? And if so, what is the nature of the relationship between the dance experience and this entity? Certainly anorexia nervosa is currently receiving much attention—both in the lay press and in the medical literature—and appears to be increasing in incidence (though some observers feel that greater recognition of the entity is responsible for its seeming upsurge). In any event, let us briefly overview anorexia nervosa in fairly general terms, and then consider it from a dance perspective.

THE "RELENTLESS PURSUIT OF THINNESS"

The young woman at Over-Haden . . .
began (as her mother says) to lose her
appetite in December last, and had lost it
quite in March following: insomuch as
that for the last six months she has not
eaten or drunk anything at all, but only
wets her lips with a feather dipt in water.
—Thomas Hobbes, in a letter from Chats-
worth, October 20, 1668

Miss K. R., age fourteen, had been a plump, healthy girl until the
beginning of 1887, at which point she began, "without apparent

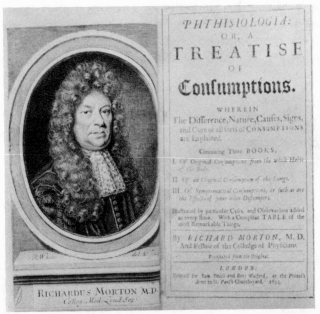

Figure 12: Frontispiece of *Phthisiologia: or, a Treatise of Consumptions*, in which
   Richard Morton is credited with the first description of anorexia nervosa
   in the medical literature. The affliction of Mr. Duke's eighteen-year-old
   daughter was termed a nervous atrophy, or *Atrophia vel Phthisis nervosa*.
(Courtesy of the Logan Clendening History of Medicine Library, the University of Kansas
Medical Center)

cause, to evince a repugnance to food; and soon afterwards declined to take any whatever, except half a cup of tea or coffee." By the time she visited the house of Sir William Gull, physician to Guy's Hospital in London, on April 20, she was extremely emaciated, so much so as to be an object of remark to passers-by as she walked through the streets. For a height of five feet four inches, she weighed only 63 pounds. Her extremities were blue and cold, her pulse somewhat slow (46), and her temperature slightly below the normal standard (97 degrees). Nonetheless, physical examination showed no signs of organic disease, and the patient "expressed herself as quite well."[66] (see figure 13).

The case of Miss K. R., which appeared in the March 17, 1888, issue of *The Lancet,* was the last contribution to the study of clinical medicine by Sir William. The case report of anorexia nervosa was an appropriate coda for the physician who had coined the term fourteen years earlier in the *Transactions of the Clinical Society,* stressing the loss of appetite (anorexia) rather

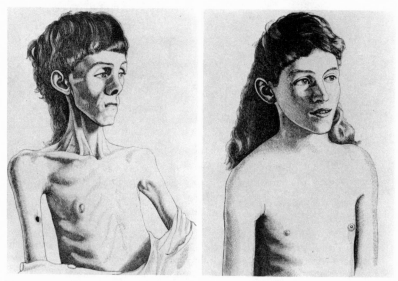

Figure 13: Before and after engravings of Miss K. R., first seen by Sir William Gull in April, 1887, and reported as a case history of anorexia nervosa in the *Lancet,* March 17, 1888.

than the pronounced loss of flesh. Sir William believed the want of appetite to be due to a "morbid mental state," since the fact "that mental states may destroy appetite is notorious, and it will be admitted that young women at the ages named are especially obnoxious to mental perversity."[67] Incidentally, the two case histories presented in 1874, as well as that of Miss K. R., culiminated in recovery, though mention was made of a case with a fatal termination.

Since its classical description by Gull, anorexia nervosa has remained an enigma to medicine, as reflected by the voluminous literature concerning this "rare" syndrome. The confusion of our predecessors as well as the difficulties encountered by current investigators in part stem from the complex and dynamic nature of the disorder. Symptoms referable to the psychological components of the problem are intermingled with those that result from nutritional deprivation. We have seen in previous chapters how simple weight loss per se may account for various body changes, such as cessation of menstruation. In the physiological sense, the same basic mechanisms may be operating in anorexia nervosa, though to a more severe extent. Excessively rigid control over eating may ultimately result in a symptom complex which is essentially one of starvation: amenorrhea and severe constipation, with hypotension (low blood pressure), hypothermia (low body temperature), bradycardia (slow heart rate), and hormonal changes which often include a low thyroid hormone, low gonadotropins, and elevated steroids (more specifically, corticoids).[68]

Along with the psychological factors that might serve to instigate the eating behavior are the influences upon thinking, feeling, and behavior which result from the self-induced malnutrition. Cause and effect become muddled and indistinguishable:

> When you lose that much weight—and especially after vomiting—you can't make sense out of things. I found that I couldn't do really simple things. I'd go the store and forget what I went for. That happens once in a while to people, but to me it would happen all the time. I felt like I was in a

constant state of confusion a lot of times. I got lost on the subways; I'd get on and then forget where I was going, or forget to get off and not know where I was, and be too weak to walk up the stairs and get out of the subway.

(The unidentified quotations in this section are taken from personal interviews of five women who sustained severe weight losses and generally conformed to the accepted diagnosis of anorexia nervosa. Two of the five required hospitalization at some point, and all either are, were, or aspired to be ballet dancers.)

It is erroneous to equate anorexia nervosa with simply "going overboard" on a diet. Dr. Hilde Bruch, one of the foremost experts on anorexia and other eating disorders, has referred to the "relentless pursuit of thinness."[69] More stiking than the emaciation is the irrational denial—denial of hunger, denial of being "too thin." It is both frustrating and horrifying to watch a young woman almost hellbent on starving herself to death, yet refusing to admit to any problem.

In a weird sort of way you find that you take pride in the way you look; even though you know you're getting thinner, you feel real good about it because it's one thing not too many people can do. Even though you may realize other things may be happening that aren't good from your weight loss, you still feel like you're rising above everybody else.

Denial of hunger implies that the term anorexia nervosa is actually a misnomer; rather than a true anorexia, or loss of appetite, the anorexic is preoccupied and constantly obsessed with food. Anorexics are often excellent cooks, forcing their creations on others but refusing to partake themselves. An all-consuming preoccupation with food, typified by such eccentric manifestations as food hoarding, ritualistic eating habits, and excessive binging followed by purging with laxatives or vomiting, is termed anorectic behavior, and appears similar to behavior patterns common to all starvation victims.

When you get that far into the whole thing, you feel guilty about almost anything you put into your mouth. If I would eat a potato chip or something, I would go to the bathroom and make myself vomit. Or if I'd eat a couple of carrot sticks. I'd really want the food so bad—I was so hungry—but I felt like I just couldn't let myself have it. I'd also chew food up and spit it out, so people around me would think I was eating. You learn a lot of little tricks like that, like hiding food under things on your plate, like lettuce.

Another aspect of behavior that is seen in many anorexics is hyperactivity, which seems even more pronounced in light of the emaciation. Sir William Gull had remarked on this aspect in his case descriptions of 1874; Miss A (5'5", 82 pounds) "was restless and active. This was, in fact, a striking expression of the nervous state, for it seemed hardly possible that a body so wasted could undergo the exercise which seemed agreeable." Concerning the second case, Miss B, he observed: "Notwithstanding the great emaciation and apparent weakness, there was a peculiar restlessness, difficult I was informed, to control. The mother added 'She is never tired.' "

I took two modern classes in the morning—which are pretty strenuous, and then would walk across Central Park over to the West Side to take a two-hour ballet class, and then walk back home again. Sometimes I'd stop on the way home to swim laps—I'd get in and swim lap after alp after lap after lap; my muscles would start cramping, and I literally could not stand up when I got out of the pool. I was blacking out from not having the energy to go on.

The following quotation conveys a sense not only of the extent of hyperactivity, distortion, and obsession concerning the body, but also of the difficulties that may be encountered early in treatment:

When I went into the hospital my weight went even lower. They were trying to put me on a special kind of diet, and I would throw away a lot of the food, order salads instead of what they put on the menu . . . I also decided that I couldn't get enough exercise in the hospital, so I'd close my door and do a special exercise class on the floor . . . and then I'd sneak out of my room and run up and down the stairs—about twelve flights of stairs—as many times as I could. I mean, I don't remember what was the most times—probably twenty times—but it would take me a good forty-five minutes to an hour to do the stairs. That's running, up and down, as fast as I could; the whole time marking up at the top on the fire extinguisher box how many times I had been up there. [Unable to keep track of the number of times, she had made hash marks on the dusty box with her finger and saliva.]

For those who have had little exposure to the problem, the presence of an anorexic can be quite disconcerting. The situation is even more difficult for family and close friends, since pleading and reasoning are of no avail to one who can't "see" realistically, who, regardless of the degree of thinness, is looking into a "fat" mirror. Because of this, anorexics become isolated and self-absorbed, avoided by acquaintances, who feel strained and uncomfortable in their presence, and often alienated from and antagonized by well-intentioned loved ones.

I was really lonely. Because if you're around people, you have to eat . . . so I would make up excuses: to have to go home, or have to shower, or have to do something, to avoid mealtime. And people don't really enjoy being around you that much either. I know I got on people's nerves just to be around; and they'd be embarrassed about wanting to eat because I wouldn't be hungry or wouldn't eat, or even worse, I would convince everybody to break their diets and go for ice cream, and then I would just take a bite. I wouldn't blame them if they hated me.

The rigid control over eating and excessive concern with the body are not themselves the problem; rather, they are symptoms of underlying factors. According to Dr. Bruch, the "relentless pursuit of thinness" is in itself a late symptom reflecting three pre-illness features of altered psychological functioning: 1) severe disturbances in body image; 2) disturbance in the accuracy of perceiving or recognizing body states, such as failing to recognize nutritional needs; and 3) an underlying sense of ineffectiveness, a conviction of helplessness in changing one's life.[70]

> I think the whole problem comes down to feeling that forces outside of you are making you do this; that you aren't doing it to yourself. You feel like other people are making you do things all the time; you feel out of control with everything in your life, except your body. And this rigid sort of dieting/exercise thing is ultimate proof of your strict control over yourself, control over your eating and not eating.

PATTERNS AND PARALLELS

> To know what kind of a person has a disease is as essential as to know what kind of a disease a person has.
> —Francis Scott Smyth

Statistically, anorexia nervosa is most prevalent among adolescent girls from "stable" middle- and upper-class families (it is extremely uncommon among males and blacks). The parents are usually self-assured, the mother often a woman of achievement (or career woman frustrated in her aspirations), the father typically successful, preoccupied with outer appearances, and admiring fitness, beauty, and achievement. The families are seemingly well functioning, but tend to gloss over or deny conflict and have difficulty adapting to stressful circumstances. The children themselves are characteristically over-achievers and "strivers," "never-give-any-trouble" children who are judgmental and who demand that others live up to the rigid value system by which they function. They may be socially isolated and overly concerned with being found wanting or not living up to expectations. Often the onset of weight loss is associated with the confronting of new experiences, in which the adolescent is faced with some changes or demands with which she is ill prepared to cope.[71]

Comparing the prototype for anorexia nervosa with the aspiring dancer in classical ballet suggests a number of uncanny parallels. To begin with, both populations consist primarily of adolescent girls. As a New York psychiatrist notes: "Many of these girls [ballet students] are getting into or going through puberty; their bodies are changing at precisely the time when demands are being made on them to really control their bodies; when there's a known upsurge in eating desire—adolescents eat more—and where problems in self-esteem and self-confidence are characteristic of the developmental age. So you've got a lot of influences all operating at the same time."

Not unusually, a young girl encouraged to study dance comes from a middle- or upper-class home, where high value is placed on achievement and on artistic pursuits, and where money is available to finance them. Once the student decides to pursue a dance career seriously, the encouragement and sacrifices required of the family may be considerable. This family support, along with the maternal "I want you to have all the opportunities I never had" may also entail considerable expectations; the frustrated mother who "lives through her children" sacrifices with strings attached. In this way, the "anorexic mother" may be sadly reminiscent of the stereotypical stage mom, putting additional demands on her progeny, imparting to them a concern about not living up to expectations, a fear of being a disappointment to the parents. A dance teacher and choreographer observes: "A lot of these kids are not dancing really because they want to dance, they're dancing because they're being pushed by mothers. Which is fine—I mean, sometimes you need to be pushed—but a lot of times it's so artificial. And then if the child doesn't get a scholarship, then she's no good, and they go through the whole thing that they won't let the kid dance if they have to pay for it and then the kid feels that she's failed."

As has been abundantly illustrated, the dance world is characterized not only by exhausting physical exercise, but also by the necessity for control, by the striving for artistic and technical proficiency, and by the overwhelming emphasis placed on the fashionable "look" and the consequent preoccupation with the body. The young dancer coming to New York to pursue a career in dance will face other changes and demands that are also challenging and stressful, pressures that have nothing to do with competition and the need for attainment of a level of professional competency. A company ballet school administrator is sympathetic: "When we speak of the young dancers coming to New York for the first time, living in residences, living in apartments, having to struggle financially; this becomes a tremendous burden, many taking jobs after classes. It's so hard, it's so sad." Another such administrator gives an idea of what's expected: "The fourteen-year-olds have academic school at 8:30, one or two subjects; they run home for [dance] class until 12:00. At 12:00 they run back to Performing Children's School where they eat something in the cafeteria, then they have academic subjects again until 2:00. At 2:00 they run like crazy, come back here, and have a [dance] class. And after that they may or may not have another [dance] class at 5:30 to 7:00, and they still have their homework to do."

In pointing out the potential similarities between the prototypical "anorexic" environment and the dance environment, I am not insinuating that the dance subculture directly causes anorexia nervosa; there is little evidence to suggest that any cultural factors are directly related to the pathogenesis of this disorder. The implications, however, are two-fold. I quote a New York City psychiatrist who has worked extensively with this disorder: "I would think that in the kind of person vulnerable or predisposed to anorexia, dancing is the kind of experience that is likely to bring out that vulnerability or predisposition. [A dancer is] so into [her] body, so attuned and sensitive to her body, that somebody whose own body image is precarious to begin with is obviously going to be much more vulnerable to the situation than somebody who has gone into a more cerebral field." And concerning the second possible relationship: "Certainly, one would expect that people with some of the characteristics of anorexia might go into dancing. By that, I mean, we know anorexics tend to be hyperactive; we know that they are very much into their bodies; we also know that they're strivers, people who want to accomplish things. And fourth, these are not only people who are strivers, but they are people who have some talent. Given a fifth ingredient; namely, some early exposure to the dance, or family influence in the dance, it's not surprising that they may move in the direction of the dance."

The empirical observation that anorexia nervosa is overrepresented in the dance population has recently been shown statistically by two Canadian researchers. The Eating Attitudes Test, an objective questionnaire highly predictive of anorexia group membership, was administered to a group of dance students, patients of comparable age with anorexia nervosa, and a control population of university students. The results are shown in Figure 14, revealing that the mean score on the test of the dancers was intermediate between the control and anorexic group, with 5 percent anorexia nervosa diagnosed among the dancers. The conclusions reached are consistent with the hypothesis just stated:

> These data support the hypothesis that individuals who focus increased emphasis on body size are at risk of anorexia nervosa and related dieting problems and that cultural variables may play a significant role in interacting with psychobiological forces in the development of anorexia nervosa in vulnerable adolescents. These findings are also compatible with the possibility that anorexic individuals may selectively enter dance schools or that high performance expectations per se rather than augmented focus on body size may facilitate the development of the syndrome.[72]

This report appeared as a letter to the editor of *The Lancet* on September 23, 1978, 104 years after Sir William Gull's classical description of anorexia nervosa in the same medical journal.

DRAWING THE LINE

> Physicians think they do a lot for a patient when they give his disease a name.
>
> —Immanuel Kant (1724–1804)

> We don't have a high percentage of that [anorexia] around here; we have people who are naturally thin—*very* thin. And

FIGURE 14

E.A.T. SCORES AND PREVALENCE OF ANOREXIA NERVOSA

Group	No.	Mean age (S.D.)	Mean E.A.T. score	Score symptomatic of anorexia*	Primary anorexia nervosa
Anorexia nervosa	33	22.5 (7.0)	58.9	33 (100%)	33
Controls	59	21.8 (2.8)	15.6	4 (7%)	0
Dance students	112	20.2 (3.3)	25.5	31 (28%)	6

*As defined by a score of 32 or greater on the eating attitudes test.[1]

The Lancet, vol. 2 , 1978, p. 674. Reproduced by permission.

some of them I really stay on their tail to keep enough food in their bodies while they're working; you know, not to be too tired and forget to eat.

—Company Ballet School Instructor

The diagnosis of anorexia nervosa is based on various criteria such as those of Feighner (see figure 15), an aggregate of characteristics constituting the typical picture established on the basis of empirical and statistical evidence. Defining a syndrome (a collection of symptoms) is necessary for making a diagnosis as well as for gathering a population for study, but the criteria are by no means absolute; in part they are subjective and in other ways arbitrary when objective (in that some "cutoff points" are necessary for definition purposes, such as "age of onset under twenty-five").

We should recognize that criteria based upon the general population may be somewhat slanted against dancers. Certainly many young ballet students in New York City 1) attain or maintain a weight significantly below standard (the standards are based on the average woman, not the average ballet dancer); 2) evidence a pattern of behavior aimed at inducing weight loss (constant dieting); 3) admit an aversion to regaining a normal weight (a "normal" weight is not an appropriate "dancing" weight); and 4) do not have menstrual periods (in my survey previously mentioned, 34 percent of the ballet students had not

From *Lancet*, September 23, 1978

Figure 15: Feighner Criteria for the diagnosis of Anorexia Nervosa

Anorexia Nervosa.—For a diagnosis of anorexia nervosa, *A* through *E* are required.

A. Age of onset prior to 25.

B. Anorexia with accompanying weight loss of at least 25% of original body weight.

C. A distorted, implacable attitude towards eating, food, or weight that overrides hunger, admonitions, reassurance and threats; eg. (1) Denial of illness with a failure to recognize nutritional needs, (2) apparent enjoyment in losing weight with overt manifestation that food refusal is a pleasurable indulgence, (3) a desired body image of extreme thinness with overt evidence that it is rewarding to the patient to achieve and maintain this state, and (4) unusal hoarding or handling of food.

D. No known medical illness that could account for the anorexia and weight loss.

E. No other known psychiatric disorder with particular reference to primary affective disorders, schizophrenia, obsessive-compulsive and phobic neurosis. (The assumption is made that even though it may appear phobic or obsessional, food refusal alone is not sufficient to qualify for obsessive-compulsive or phobic disease.)

F. At least two of the following manifestations. (1) Amenorrhea. (2) Lanugo. (3) Bradycardia (persistent resting pulse of 60 or less) (4) Periods of overactivity. (5) Episodes of bulimia. (6) Vomiting (may be self-induced).

From *Arch Gen Psychiat* 1972, 26:57, copyright 1972, American Medical Association had periods for three months or more).

So how does one classify the eighteen-year-old ballet student who is obsessed with her "look," who may abuse laxatives or induce vomiting, and considers herself "obese" at any weight over a hundred pounds? I have referred to a number of young dancers who manifest these characteristics, who are very thin by almost any standards (except their own), and who even drop to lower body weights. Nonetheless, an important distinction differentiates most from the "classical" anorexic; namely, the presence of a safety valve, the absence of the irrational denial. Perhaps, one could argue, it is a matter of the degree to which they "see" unrealistically. At some point they become frightened, don't like the way they look, or notice a loss of strength that is detrimental to their dancing. Often the weight loss is initiated as a consequence of an increased dancing schedule (such as a move to New York), a career opportunity (a crash diet of Tab and bubble gum for three days prior to an audition), poor eating habits (residence hall food is not as good as mom's; often there are no kitchen facilities and inadequate funds for eating out), or outright unrealistic demands.

> . . . a couple of summers ago I probably had a mild case of anorexia. I had a bowl of bran in the morning, and that was it for the whole day, for a whole summer. Because my director sort of brainwashed me that I was obese (I was like I am now—five-feet-two-inches, 95 pounds) and he wanted me to look like a toothpick. He sort of brainwashed me so I didn't know how far I was going. I got to about 80 pounds.
> —Ballet scholarship student

In light of the extreme example of anorexia nervosa, we must not be misled by the authoritativeness implicit in medical terminology. The need to define terms has its drawbacks as well as its limitations, and may lead to more ambiguities concerning an entity which is elusive to begin with. Classification is no easy task for the gray area between the "weight-conscious" dieter and the one who becomes self-destructive. One description which has come into usage is "thin fat people," referring to those persons who succeed in keeping their weight close to or below normal, but whose lives are centered upon the maintenance of this low weight, and who tend to interpret a slight weight gain as gross fatness. Perhaps this particular group of dancers might be termed "pseudo-anorexic," "anorexoid," or simply possessing "anorectic" behavior. One New York psychiatrist experienced with dancers felt uncomfortable with any reference implying anorexia nervosa and spoke simply of "neurotic excesses." These excesses may be learned or conditioned, and may even have survival value in the current dance subculture. What appears as a "mild" anorexic syndrome may not necessarily have as a basis the same dynamics or implications as the classical syndrome and may exist in a person who is reasonably well functioning personally as well as professionally.

Regardless of the terminology one prefers, a very significant problem in the dance world is the recognition of potentially dangerous eating disorders; psychological disturbances of the severity of anorexia nervosa are crippling and life-threatening, and professional help must be sought before a chronic state develops. Not only are anorexia nervosa and similar problems more prevalent in the dance world, but in the midst of "naturally thin" women, dancers with problems may be well camouflaged. "Drawing the line" is never easy, but it is especially crucial that dance teachers, choreographers, administrators, and dancers themselves be aware of, and responsive to, problems of this nature. Too often the "line" is determined on a purely visual basis, as in the case of the ballet scholarship student who says: "It's different for everybody. Each body looks differently; but I find it when a person is too thin to complete a graceful line, where the body gets to the point where it's angular instead of curved. When you look at the person and they don't look pleasing, that's the point."

As far as criteria go, the above isn't particularly accurate or sensitive. One must be more mindful of behavior, of attitudes toward body and self. The "look," for obvious reasons, simply doesn't make it as a standard.

Beyond the Mirror

Let me describe one of my favorite dancers, whom I shall call Cindy, and who just turned thirteen years old. Cindy is a mature, intelligent, and beautiful young woman with a variety of talents and interests. Although she enjoys ballet, she has doubts about making it a career; she only takes a maximum of two or three ballet classes per week, while emphasizing gymnastics training during the summer months. Most of Cindy's close friends are not dancers, but are classmates at a public junior high school. Cindy eats well, is a top student, and has a secure family relationship. Not surprisingly, she has never had a weight problem, weighing in at about eighty-five pounds. In short, Cindy is about the healthiest little girl I know.

Cindy was accepted in a summer dance program in New York City, and I was privileged to have her as a houseguest for a month. The experience was quite a revelation. In the "real ballet world," the girls were a different breed from most of her friends at home, not just in their seriousness and dedication to the dance, but mainly in their acceptance of restrictions and limitations in their life styles. This was a bit discouraging to my friend, who had a lot of life exploring to do and didn't feel immediately pressed into making career decisions (especially with two full years left in junior high). But for a month she danced, and enjoyed her dancing, and I can't help but think that this healthy little girl also had a very healthy attitude toward dance for a thirteen-year-old.

On the last day of the program, Cindy was given an oral evaluation. Surprised that she didn't rush to tell me what was said, and assuming her reluctance would have modesty as its basis, I asked her outright.

"How was your evaluation?"

"It was all right," she said, somewhat subdued.

"What did she say?"

"She said that I was a very strong dancer."

"That's terrific. What else?"

"That's about all."

"That was it?"

"Pretty much, except that she also told me I had to watch my weight." Saying this, her eyes began to tear.

I was dumbstruck. The simple criticism took on magnified proportions as a minute trauma—that, compounded with similar others,—could potentially have a very negative effect on an adolescent's formation of attitudes about body and self-image. To begin with, Cindy did not have a weight problem; the problem was a distorted standard of perception. But supposing, for argument's sake, that she was five pounds too heavy. Might not the criticism still be unwarranted, a needless cruelty? What professional demands could preclude an adolescent, approaching the peak of her growth spurt, from carrying this minimal additional weight? Are five pounds really an issue in this case, worth the risk of imposing guilt, fostering a sense of inadequacy, and compounding the pressures of developing technique and succeeding as a dancer?

"That's ridiculous," I said. "You feel all right?"

"Not very good." She paused and took a deep breath, doing her best to control that accumulation of fluid precariously balanced within her lower eyelid.

"Do you think you're overweight?"

"No," she answered confidently, then added, "well, maybe for a dancer . . ."

"Come on, now, be honest."

"I don't think so."

I asked her what she had done after receiving the evaluation and she shrugged. I asked her about lunch, and she informed me that she had eaten at Amy's, where she had her customary salad.

And how did she feel about lunch? She felt very full afterwards, and guilty about eating the entire plate. But wasn't that odd? She almost always had the same salad when she went to Amy's, and she always emptied the bowl, and she had never felt exceptionally full or guilty about it previously.

It remains to be seen what significance this minor incident

may have; perhaps it represents nothing more than a ballet administrator's putting a damper on a girl's lunch. When I had an opportunity to interview the school administrator a few weeks later, any anger that I still felt dissipated as soon as she spoke. The truth was that there was no one specifically toward whom I could direct any anger.

She pointed out initially that she was simply the administrator, delivering the evaluations given to her by the teachers. She also did not feel that telling a little girl to "watch her weight" was particularly harsh, though she admitted that some of the girls "tend to be oversensitive" about their weight and that even mild criticism "for them, apparently . . . is too much." Besides, she said, "watch your weight" is just a general comment, one that applies to nearly every dancer. It's almost a throwaway criticism: a little girl asks, "What do I improve on?" and a simple reply is "Watch your weight," much as one would advise adequate sleep and good eating to stay healthy. There was also another very reasonable and realistic justification.

"You cannot stop in time, you have to look to the future," she told me. "That same little girl . . . is going to reaudition for next summer, because she wants to come back, she did a good job, and she is proud of having been here. . . . If this little girl—having not been told anything—as you say has a growth spurt and is eating . . . all of a sudden this little girl is not taken back. Then you face another terrible emotional crisis a year later. And you see, I think you have to balance that; we are concerned about that, too. And it's worse. All right, maybe she was unhappy one day, but having thought about it probably said, 'Well, you know, "watch your weight" is not terribly serious.' It's terrible for these kids if they come to us one year and the next year they are rejected [because of weight]."

A teacher who ignores a weight problem is without question failing in her obligation to prepare a student for the realities of a career in dance. But many factors are involved, and sensitivity to individual needs and situations is essential. For example, discussing weight privately with a fourteen-year-old is different from browbeating her in class and embarrassing her among her peers. A student may also react differently to such admonitions, depending on her own ability, competition, pressures, whether she lives at home with parents or in a residence hall with dancers, etc. And a sixteen-year-old who is overweight may actually have more of a problem than a ten-year-old with "baby fat" who hasn't hit her growth spurt.

In the weight-obsessive dance subculture, those who pass judgment on weight may well be overzealous and their expectations unrealistic. The burden, however, whether it is needless or not, ultimately falls on the youngsters—the least defended, most vulnerable, and most impressionable. The psychological ramifications are difficult to assess, but the fact that some young dancers routinely practice laxative and diuretic abuse and self-induced vomiting leads one to suspect that the scars may be more than physiological.

The dance subculture is a stressful and difficult environment for all concerned, and as a model, it provides a valuable lesson. If unforeseen circumstances like those I have outlined result from maintaining a dancing weight that for some may be unphysiologic, the blame can only be laid diffusely. The major culprit is the distortion of body image that permeates nearly every aspect of our society—the dance world is simply allotted a larger and more conspicuous dose of it.

Over the past few months I have witnessed my own subtle transformation as part of the dance audience: more often now am I distracted uncomfortably by an angular line of a dancer who is too thin. And a common question—"Wouldn't it be better to be five pounds too light than five pounds too heavy?"—which I once answered overwhelmingly in the affirmative, elicits a different response. To begin with, five pounds either way doesn't seem to warrant the concern of a national emergency. And second, since emaciation and morbid obesity are equally undesirable extremes, lesser gradations don't particularly tip the scale one way or the other.

To modify our aesthetic sensibilities may take a conscious,

individual effort; we should not depend on the arts or fashion to help us adjust our vision. The change need not be drastic or accomplished overnight; it might be as subtle as the visual adjustments that have gradually brought us to our present perspective. Consider a more deliberate look at the *Venus de Milo,* disregarding for a moment the fashion shows, the magazine spreads, the display window mannequins. Actually, you may think, if she were decked out in the right outfit, she might not look so bad after all.

Notes

1. For glimpses of the dance experience in professional ballet companies, see: S. Forsyth and P. M. Kolenda, "Competition, Cooperation, and Group Cohesion in the Ballet Company," *Psychiatry* 29 (1966): 123–45; J. H. Mazo, *Dance Is a Contact Sport* (New York: Da Capo Press, 1974); F. Stevens, *Dance As Life: A Season with American Ballet Theatre* (New York: Harper & Row, 1976).

2. Many dancers enhance the usually short lifespan of pointe shoes by hardening them with multiple applications of clear acrylic floor wax.

3. J. A. Nicholas, "Risk Factors in Sports Medicine and the Orthopedic System: An Overview," *Journal of Sports Medicine* 3 (1976): 243–59.

4. ––*Employment and Unemployment of Artists: 1970–1975*, National Endowment for the Arts Research Division Report no. 1 (April 1976).

5. A. de Mille, *Dance to the Piper* (Boston: Little, Brown & Co., 1952), p. 54.

6. Information furnished by the public relations department, National Football League.

7. Information furnished by the New York City Ballet.

8. Informal survey of members of the Martha Graham Company.

9. From Balanchine-Gruen interview in J. Gruen, *The Private World of Ballet* (New York: Penguin, 1975), p. 282.

10. F. Heckel, *Les grandes et petites obésités* (Paris: Masson et Cie, 1911), as quoted in H. Bruch, *Eating Disorders: Obesity, Anorexia Nervosa, and the Person Within* (New York: Basic Books, 1973) p. 18–19.

11. B. Rudofsky, *The Unfashionable Human Body* (New York: Doubleday, Anchor Press, 1974), p. 189.

12. For a fascinating account of the history of tuberculosis, from which much of the material on consumption and the Romantic age is derived, see: R. Dubos and J. Dubos, *The White Plague* (Boston: Little, Brown & Co., 1952).

13. From the memoirs of Alexandre Dumas, as quoted in Dubos and Dubos, *The White Plague*, p. 59.

14. O. Fischel and M. von Boehn, *Modes and Manners of the Nineteenth Century as Represented in the Pictures and Engravings of the Time*, trans. M. Edwards (New York: E. P. Dutton & Co., 1909), vol. 2, p. 149.

15. J. Burnett, *Plenty and Want: A Social History of Diet in England from 1815 to the Present Day* (London: Thomas Nelson and Sons, 1966), p. 56–57.

16. V. Bullough and M. Voght, "Women, Menstruation, and Nineteenth-Century Medicine," *Bulletin of the History of Medicine* 47 (1973): 66–82.

17. Dubos and Dubos, *The White Plague*, p. 247.

18. For additional insight into the health dilemmas of these nineteenth-century maidens, see: R. P. Hudson, "The Biography of Disease: Lessons from Chlorosis," *Bulletin of the History of Medicine* 51 (1977): 448–63; E. P. Scarlett, "Doctor Out of Zebulun: The Vapors," *Archives of Internal Medicine* 116 (July 1965): 142–46.

19. P. Miguel, *The Ballerinas—From the Court of Louis XIV to Pavlova* (New York: Macmillan Co., 1972), p. 216.

20. G. Carson, *Cornflake Crusade* (New York: Rinehart and Co., 1957), p. 50.

21. For a review of energy storage and use as it relates to fasting, see: G. F. Cahill, "Starvation in Man," *New England Journal of Medicine* 282 (1970): 668–75.

22. P. Felig and J. Wahren, "Fuel Homeostasis in Exercise," *New England Journal of Medicine* 293 (1975): 1078–84.

23. For an excellent and more comprehensive review on the physiology of insulin, see: G. F. Cahill, "Physiology of Insulin in Man," *Diabetes* 20 (December 1971): 785–99.

24. Although genuine hypoglycemia with exercise is uncommon, it has been observed in marathon runners and in patients on low carbohydrate diets. I am aware of no studies of this type dealing exclusively with dancers, but it would seem likely that strenuous dancing combined with a semistarvation carbohydrate regimen and low body fat stores could eventuate in actual hypoglycemia in some instances.

25. B. N. Park et al., "Insulin-Glucose Dynamics in Nondiabetic Reactive Hypoglycemia and Asymptomatic Biochemical Hypoglycemia in Normals, Prediabetics, and Chemical Diabetics, " *Diabetes* 21 (1972): 273.

26. T. J. Merimee and J. E. Tyson, "Stabilization of Plasma Glucose during Fasting: Normal Variations in Two Separate Studies," *New England Journal of Medicine* 291 (1974): 1275-77.

27. See C. K. Meador, "The Art and Science of Nondisease," *New England Journal of Medicine* 272 (1965): 92-95; G. F. Cahill and J. S. Soeldner, "A Non-editorial on Nonhypoglycemia," ibid. 291 (1974): 905-906; J. Yager and R. T. Young, "Non-Hypoglycemia Is an Epidemic Condition," ibid. 907-908; F. D. Hofeldt et al., "Postprandial Hypoglycemia: Fact or Fiction?" *Journal of the American Medical Association* 233 (1975): 1309.

28. A. H. Crisp, "The Possible Significance of Some Behavioral Correlates of Weight and Carbohydrate Intake," *Journal of Psychosomatic Research* 11 (1967): 117-31.

29. Reported in E. R. Novak et al., *Textbook of Gynecology*, 8th ed. (Baltimore: Williams and Wilkins Co., 1970)

30. M. H. Williams, *Nutritional Aspects of Human Physical and Athletic Performance* (Springfield, Ill.: Charles C. Thomas, 1976), p. 177.

31. K. A. Smiles and S. Robinson, "Sodium Ion Conservation during Acclimatization of Men to Work in the Heat," *Journal of Applied Physiology* 31 (1971): 63-69; D. L. Costill et al., "Water and Electrolyte Replacement during Repeated Days of Work in the Heat," *Aviation, Space, and Environmental Medicine*, June 1975, pp. 795-800.

32. T. B. Van Itallie and M. Yang, "Current Concepts in Nutrition: Diet and Weight Loss," *New England Journal of Medicine* 297 (1977): 1158-61.

33. Ibid.

34. D. L. Costill, "The Drinking Runner," in *The Complete Diet Guide for Runners and Other Athletes*, ed. Hal Higdon (Mountain View, Calif.: World Publications, 1978), pp. 151-67.

35. For examples of some of the ramifications of self-abusive practices, see: J. de Graeff and M. A. M. Schuurs, "Severe Potassium Depletion Caused by the Abuse of Laxatives: One Patient Followed for Eight Years," *Acta Medica Scandinavica* 166 (1960): 407-22; H. P. Wolff et al., "Psychiatric Disturbance Leading to Potassium Depletion, Sodium Depletion, Raised Plasma-Renin Concentration, and Secondary Hyperaldosteronism," *Lancet* 1 (1968): 258-61.

36. G. Majno, *The Healing Hand* (Cambridge: Harvard University Press, 1975), p. 129.

37. A. Abrahams, *The Human Machine* (Harmondsworth, Middlesex: Penguin Books, 1956), pp. 104-107.

38. From A. J. Ryan and F. L. Allman, eds., *Sports Medicine* (New York: Academic Press, 1974), p. 17.

39. A. Castiglioni, *A History of Medicine*, trans. E. B. Krumbhaar (New York; Alfred A. Knopf 1941), p. 1754.

40. L. S. Goodman and A. Gilman, eds., *The Pharmacological Basis of Therapeutics*, 5th ed. (New York: Macmillan Co., 1975), p. 982.

41. A. de Mille, *And Promenade Home* (Boston: Little, Brown & Co., 1958), p. 224.

42. J. V. Ricci, *The Genealogy of Gynaecology: History of the Development of Gynaecology throughout the Ages* (Philadelphia: Blakiston Co., 1943), p. 194.

43. Dancing, Hippocrates believed, is beneficial for amenorrhea, as well as useful for inducing abortion.

44. J. V. Ricci, *One Hundred Years of Gynaecology: 1800–1900* (Philadelphia: Blakiston Co., 1945), p. 519.

45. Ibid., p. 521.

46. J. Whitehead, *On the Causes and Treatment of Abortion and Sterility* (Philadelphia: Lea & Blanchard, 1848), p. 61.

47. R. E. Frisch and R. Revelle, "Height and Weight at Menarche and a Hypothesis of Menarche," *Archives of Disease in Childhood* 46 (1971): 695–701.

48. R. E. Frisch and J. W. McArthur, "Menstrual Cycles: Fatness as a Determinant of Minimum Weight for Height Necessary for Their Maintenance or Onset," *Science* 185 (1974): 949–51.

49. R. E. Frisch, "A Method of Prediction of Age of Menarche from Height and Weight at Ages Nine through Thirteen Years," *Pediatrics* 53 (1974): 384–90.

50. Frisch and McArthur, "Menstrual Cycles."

51. C. Darwin, *The Variation of Animals and Plants under Domestication* (London: John Murray, 1868), vol. 2, p. 112.

52. Some of the data concerning this subject is unpublished. In a personal communication to the author, Dr. Harmon Brown, director of Student Health Services at California State University at Hayward, reported a study of twenty runners. Four (between the ages of fifteen and seventeen) had primary amenorrhea, and another four had secondary amenorrhea when they trained intensively. Correspondence with Ken Foreman, director of education and research at the Northwest Sports Medicine Foundation, revealed that approximately 40 percent of their female distance runners encounter amenorrhea.

53. From M. Albohm, "Does Menstruation Affect Performance in Sports?" *The Physician and Sportsmedicine,* March 1976, pp. 76–78.

54. I heard this originally from two different Russian ballet dancers; it was confirmed by a physician associated with ballet in Russia until fairly recently.

55. R. E. Frisch, R. Revelle, and S. Cook, "Components of the Critical Weight at Menarche and at Initiation of the Adolescent Spurt: Estimated Total Water, Lean Body Mass and Fat," *Human Biology* 45 (1973): 469–83.

56. R. M. Malina et al., "Age of Menarche and Selected Menstrual Characteristics in Athletes at Different Competitive Levels and in Different Sports," *Medicine and Science in Sports* 10 (1978): 218–22.

57. R. M. Malina et al., "Age at Menarche in Athletes and Non-Athletes," *Medicine and Science in Sports* 5 (1973): 11–13.

58. R. A. Vigersky et al., "Hypothalamic Dysfunction in Secondary Amenorrhea Associated with Simple Weight Loss," *New England Journal of Medicine* 297 (1977): 1141–45.

59. E. N. Wilmsen, "Seasonal Effects of Dietary Intake on Kalahari San," *Federation Proceedings* 37 (1978): 65–72; L. A. van der Walt et al., "Unusual Sex Hormone Patterns among Desert-Dwelling Hunter-Gatherers," *Journal of Clinical Endocrinology and Metabolism* 46 (1978): 658–63.

60. C. Gopalan and A. N. Naidu, "Nutritition and Fertility," *Lancet* 2 (1972): 1077–78.

61. The congenital disorder was gonadal dysgenesis, or Turner's syndrome, the key defect being a genetic abnormality of an X chromosome.

62. Quoted in de Mille, *Dance to the Piper,* p. 65.

63. Ibid., p. 54.

64. De Mille, *And Promenade Home,* p. 227.

65. The Ballet Company: A Game for Dancers and Balletomanes of All Ages. Copyright 1973 by Lynne Stetson.

66. W. W. Gull, "Anorexia Nervosa," *Lancet,* 17 March 1888.

67. W. W. Gull, *Transactions of the Clinical Society of London* 7 (1874): 22. Sir William, in a medical address at Oxford in the fall of 1868, mentioned a "peculiar form of disease"

which he termed "apepsia hysterica." In a paper in the *Archives générales de Médecine* of April 1873, a Dr. Laségue described the malady as "hysterical anorexia." Evidently, by 1874 Sir William had, without being aware of the publication of the French journal, decided that "anorexia" was a more appropriate term. Thus, anorexia nervosa became a clinical entity almost simultaneously with the independent reports from England and France slightly more than a hundred years ago.

68. M. P. Warren and R. L. Vande Wiele, "Clinical and Metabolic Features of Anorexia Nervosa," *American Journal of Obstetrics and Gynecology* 117 (1973): 435–49.

69. See the following excellent treatments of the entity: H. Bruch, *Eating Disorders: Obesity, Anorexia Nervosa, and the Person Within* (New York: Basic Books, 1973); and Bruch, *The Golden Cage: The Enigma of Anorexia Nervosa* (Cambridge: Harvard University Press, 1978).

70. H. Bruch, "Anorexia Nervosa and Its Differential Diagnosis," *Journal of Nervous and Mental Disease* 141 (1966): 555–66.

71. In presenting this simplified portrait, I have drawn primarily from the works of Dr. Bruch and the following: S. Minuchin, B. L. Rosman, and L. Baker, *Psychosomatic Families: Anorexia Nervosa in Context* (Cambridge: Harvard University Press, 1978). Additionally, for a recent and comprehensive monograph on all aspects of anorexia nervosa, see: R. A. Vigersky, ed., *Anorexia Nervosa,* monograph of the National Institute of Child Health and Human Development (New York: Raven Press, 1977).

72. D. M. Garner and P. E. Garfinkel, "Sociocultural Factors in Anorexia Nervosa" (letter to the editor), *Lancet* 2 (1978): 674.

In a recent paper presented at the annual meeting of the American Psychiatric Association, Drs. Garner and Garfinkel updated this study. Results indicated that 44 percent of 183 female dance students displayed scores on the Eating Attitudes Test which were in the range of the anorexia nervosa patients. Twelve cases (6.5 percent) of primary anorexia nervosa were detected clinically in the dance group using rigorous diagnostic criteria.

Glossary

Adrenocorticotropin (ACTH). A pituitary hormone that stimulates the adrenal gland (more specifically, the outer layer or cortex).

Aldosterone. The principal electrolyte-regulating hormone of the adrenal gland, primarily concerned with sodium balance.

Amenorrhea. Absence or abnormal stoppage of menstrual flow; may be primary (failure of menstruation to occur at puberty) or secondary (cessation of menstruation once it has been established).

Amino Acids. The basic components of protein.

Anorexia (true). Lack or loss of appetite.

Anorexia Nervosa. A syndrome characterized by severe emaciation resulting from self-imposed weight loss.

Anti-diuretic Hormone (ADH). A hormone secreted by the pituitary gland that diminishes the amount of urine produced.

Beta Cells. The insulin-producing cells of the pancreas.

Blood Sugar. Glucose circulating in the bloodstream (the form in which carbohydrate is transported in the blood).

Bradycardia. Abnormally slow heart rate.

Bulimia. Compulsive eating of an extreme nature, usually followed by self-induced vomiting.

Carbohydrate. A group of organic compounds, including the sugars, starches, and celluloses.

Cathartic. A medicine that quickens and increases bowel evacuation.

Consumption. A wasting away of the body; antiquated terminology for tuberculosis.

Corticoid. A term applied to hormones of the outer layer, or cortex, of the adrenal gland.

Dehydration. A condition resulting from the loss of body water.

Diuresis. Increased urination.

Diuretic. An agent that promotes urination; commonly called a "water pill."

Dysmenorrhea. Pain associated with menstruation.

Electrocardiogram. A graphic tracing of the electric current produced with contraction of the heart.

Electrolytes. Referring to elements which have the property of carrying an electrical charge when dissolved in solution.

Emesis. Vomiting.

Emetic. An agent that causes vomiting.

Endometrium. The inner lining of the uterus, the structure and thickness of which varies with the phases of the menstrual cycle.

Estrogen. "Female sex hormone" with wide variety of functions, including effects on endometrium, breast growth and development, vaginal lining and secretions, and deposition of body fat.

Fatty Acids. Body fuel for low intensity exercise; along with glycerol a component of triglycerides.

Feedback. The return of the end product of a pathway or system to serve as input (either positive or negative).

Follicle (ovarian). The ovum along with the cystlike structure of surrounding cells which serves to nourish and protect the egg as it matures.

Follicular Stimulating Hormone (FSH). Pituitary hormone acting on the ovary, stimulating the growth of the ovarian follicle.

Gluconeogenesis. The formation of carbohydrate from molecules which are not themselves carbohydrate, such as protein or fat.

Glucose. A simple sugar or monosaccharide.

Glycerol. Along with fatty acids, a part of triglycerides.

Glycogen. The chief storage form of carbohydrate, in muscle and liver; used primarily in high intensity exercise.

Glycogenolysis. The breakdown of glycogen in the body.

Gonadotropins. Hormones stimulating sexual glands, two of which include FSH and LH.

Growth Hormone (GH). Pituitary hormone with wide range of effects, principal among which includes involvement with normal growth.

Growth Spurt. Developmental period characterized by rapid increase in height and weight; in the female, it begins at about age eight or nine, peaks shortly before menarche, and is virtually complete one to three years postmenarche.

Hormones. Chemical substances which have specific effects on a certain organ or "target."

Hypoglycemia. An abnormal decrease in blood sugar level.

Hypokalemia. Abnormally low potassium content in the blood.

Hyponatremia. Abnormally low sodium content in the blood.

Hypotension. Lowered blood pressure.

Hypothalamic-Pituitary-Ovarian Axis. Referring to the sum total of interrelationships involved with maintaining the integrity of female hormonal balance.

Hypothalamic Releasing Factors. Hormones of the hypothalamus that regulate hormonal production of the pituitary gland.

Hypothalamus. Section of the brain involved with, among other things, water balance, satiety, sleep, and temperature regulation.

Hypothermia. Low body termperature.

Hypothyroidism. Deficiency of thyroid activity.

Insulin. Hormone secreted by the beta cells of the pancreas concerned with the regulation of carbohydrate metabolism.

Ion. Atom or group of atoms that carry a positive or negative electrical charge.

Lactate. An end product of sugar breakdown (in the absense of oxygen).

Laxative. An agent that promotes bowel evacuation; a mild cathartic.

Luteinizing Hormone (LH). The pituitary hormone involved in the stimulation of ovulation.

Menarche. The onset of menstrual function.

Menstrual Dysfunction. Any disturbance, impairment, or abnormality of menstruation.

Menstruation. Cyclic physiologic uterine bleeding.

Metabolism. The sum total of all chemical and physical processes—constructive as well as destructive—by which a living organism is maintained.

Misattribution. The attributing of a symptom to an incorrect cause.

Oligomenorrhea. Abnormally infrequent or scanty menstruation.

Ovulation. The expulsion of a "ripe" ovarian follicle into the Fallopian tube for possible fertilization.

Pathologic. Indicative of or caused by a diseased condition.

Physiologic. Normal, not pathologic.

Physiology. The study of the function of the living organism and its parts.

Pituitary. A small gland at the base of the brain responsible for the secretion of a variety of hormones.

Placebo Effect. A diminished perception of symptoms after "treatment" with an inactive substance.

Progesterone. Hormone which functions to prepare the uterus for reception and development of a fertilized ovum by stimulating glandular proliferation of the endometrium.

Prolactin. A pituitary hormone which stimulates lactation in mammary glands.

Purgative. A cathartic.

Pyruvate. An intermediary organic substance in energy metabolism.

Steroids. A group name of compounds, included in which are the sex hormones.

Syndrome. A set of symptoms occurring together.

Thyroid Stimulating Hormone (TSH). A pituitary hormone that stimulates the thyroid gland.